INTRODUCTION

We've all heard that breakfast is the most important meal of the day. This statement is particularly true with the Ketogenic Diet. Breakfast kick starts your metabolism, helping you burn calories throughout the day. In fact, studies have shown that breakfast plays an important role in helping to maintain a healthy body weight. Starting the day with a low-carb, high-protein breakfast will leave you satiated for hours. And a breakfast free of refined sugars and carbohydrates will keep you focused and energized until lunchtime.

To help you get the most out of this diet, below are 50 of the best breakfast recipes around. The recipes are broken into two categories: Quick and Easy Weekday Recipes and Weekend/Brunch Recipes. The weekday recipes were designed with limited time in mind. Many of them are great 'make ahead' meals that you can have on hand throughout the week. The weekend recipes require a bit more cooking time and are wonderful for family breakfasts.

I hope you enjoy the recipes and they help you on your journey to a healthier you.

QUICK & EASY WEEKDAY RECIPES

WEEKEND / BRUNCH RECIPES

Adjusting and customizing the recipes

These recipes have been created to:

1. Be easy to make

2. Be delicious

3. Use easy to find ingredients

However, there is not a one-size-fits-all recipe, everyone has different tastes, some have allergies and not everyone will be able to get all of the ingredients. Consider the recipes as a guideline to which you can then customize to your taste or to what you have in the house.

» Love coconut? Try coconut flour instead of almond.

» Do not have any pink rock salt in the house? Just use some normal table salt instead.

» Do not like strawberries? Try blueberries.

» Prefer your eggs a bit runnier? Cook them for slightly less time.

» Don't want to cook 4 servings? Simply halve the ingredients and only cook 2.

I have included some suggestions throughout for alternatives, but could not list every single one. Only you know what your preferences are, so have some fun with it and play around with different ingredients and recipes.

And lastly, if you would be kind enough to leave an honest review it would be most appreciated. Please visit the link below:

http://geni.us/KetoBreakReview

Once again, thank you for downloading and good luck.

Elizabeth Jane

QUICK & EASY
WEEKDAY RECIPES

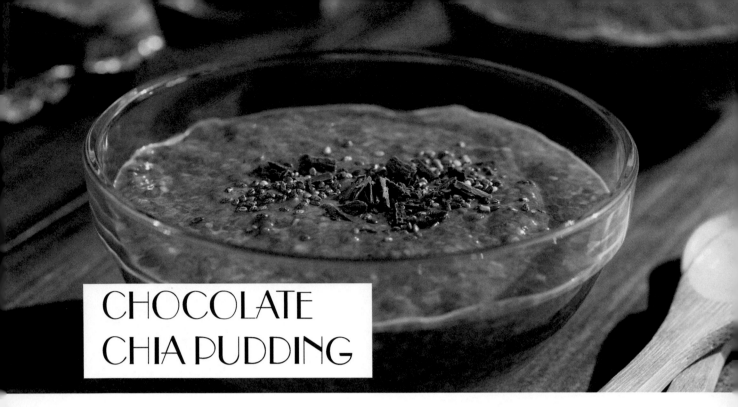

CHOCOLATE CHIA PUDDING

🥄 **2 minutes**   🕐 **3 minutes**   👤 **2**

INGREDIENTS

- » 2 tablespoons chia seeds
- » 4 scoops chocolate protein powder
- » 2 tablespoons ground flax seeds
- » ½ cup almond flour
- » 1 cup canned coconut milk
- » 4 tablespoons hemp hearts
- » ⅔ cup water
- » ¼ tablespoon ground cinnamon
- » ¼ tablespoon ground nutmeg

Suggested toppings
- » Toasted almonds
- » Toasted coconut
- » Almond butter

DIRECTIONS

1. It is better to prepare this dish the night before serving to allow the flavors to combine and the seeds and flour to absorb the liquid.
2. Combine the coconut milk and water together in a medium bowl. Combine the chia seeds, protein powder, flax seeds, almond flour, cinnamon, and nutmeg in a separate bowl.
3. Make a well in the dry ingredients and pour the milk/water mixture little by little into the dry ingredients while continuously mixing. Repeat until the ingredients are thoroughly mixed together. Cover the bowl and place in the fridge overnight.
4. The next day, place the mixture in a small saucepan and use a gentle heat. Bring the mixture to a simmer and stir frequently until it thickens. The thickness should not be too runny, but not solid either. This can be to your personal preference.
5. Stir in the hemp hearts just before serving.
6. Divide evenly between two bowls and add your favorite healthy toppings.

- - - - - - - - - - - - - -

Suggestions: Try different flavor protein powders, such as vanilla and strawberry, for different tasting results.

NUTRITION FACTS (PER SERVING)

Total Carbohydrates: 20g	Dietary Fiber: 10g	Net Carbs: 10g
Protein: 38g	Total Fat: 32g	Calories: 486

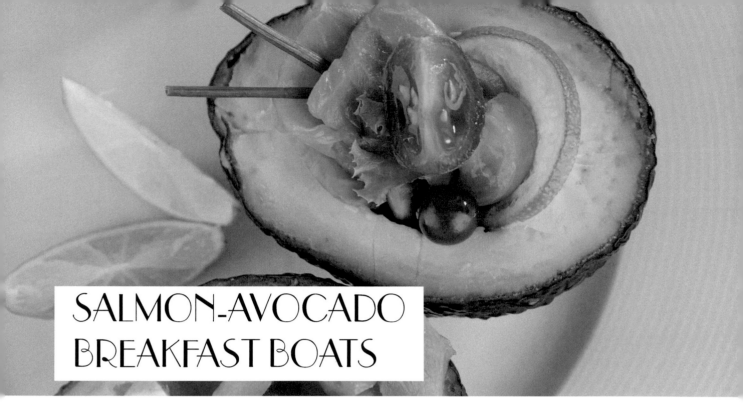

SALMON-AVOCADO BREAKFAST BOATS

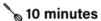 10 minutes   0 minutes   4

INGREDIENTS

» 2 ripe avocados
» 4 ounces wild-caught smoked salmon
» 8 cherry tomatoes, halved
» 2 limes, for juice and garnish
» Sea salt and pepper to taste

DIRECTIONS

1. Marinate the salmon in the juice of one lime for about an hour.
2. Cut the avocados in half lengthwise and remove the seeds.
3. Cut the salmon into thin strips and place into the avocado center.
4. Top each avocado half with a lime wedge and several cherry tomato halves.
5. Serve immediately.

Salmon is high in an omega-3 fatty acid called DHA which helps to protect against heart disease, lowers cholesterol, and may help slow Alzheimer's. In addition to that, it contains nearly 6 grams of protein per ounce!

NUTRITION FACTS (PER SERVING)

Total Carbohydrates: 4g	Dietary Fiber: 2g	Net Carbs: 2g
Protein: 10g	Total Fat: 24g	Calories: 263

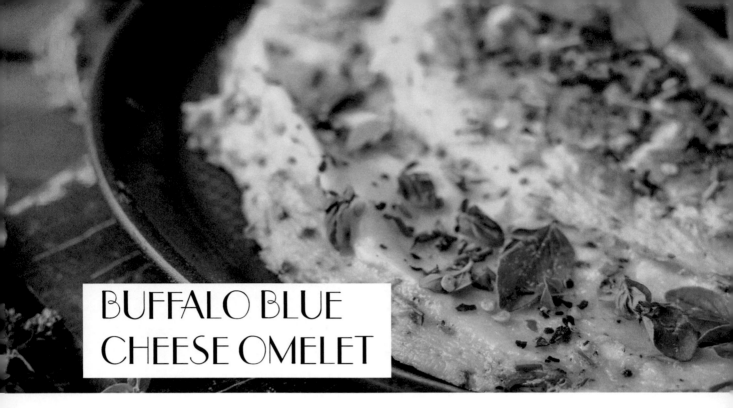

BUFFALO BLUE CHEESE OMELET

🥄 **5 minutes**   🕐 **10 minutes**   👤 **4**

INGREDIENTS

- » 4 ounces cream cheese, softened
- » 4 tablespoons blue cheese
- » 2 tablespoons hot sauce (adjust to suit your taste)
- » 6 eggs
- » 2 tablespoons water
- » 2 tablespoons coconut oil
- » Garnishes: Chopped fresh parsley and chives

DIRECTIONS

1. In a small bowl, heat the cream cheese, blue cheese, and hot sauce in the microwave for about 15 seconds. Stir until smooth and combined.
2. In a separate bowl, whisk the eggs until frothy.
3. Heat about half a tablespoon of coconut oil in a non-stick pan over medium heat. Pour one quarter of the eggs into the pan. Drop one quarter of the cream cheese mixture by spoonfuls over half of the eggs.
4. Once the eggs have firmed up, fold the empty half over the half with filling. Cover, lower heat, and allow to cook for about another minute.
5. Carefully remove from pan, cover with tin foil to keep warm, and repeat with the remaining eggs and filling.

Eggs are a very good source of inexpensive, high-quality protein. They also have impressive health credentials. The whites are rich sources of selenium and vitamin D while the yoke contains fat soluble vitamins such as A, D, E and K. So don't skip the yolk.

NUTRITION FACTS (PER SERVING)

Total Carbohydrates: 2g	Dietary Fiber: 0g	Net Carbs: 2g
Protein: 12g	Total Fat: 26g	Calories: 282

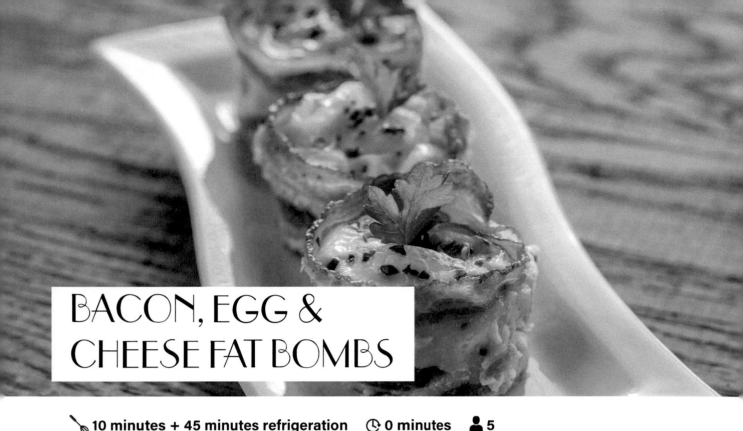

BACON, EGG & CHEESE FAT BOMBS

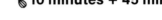 10 minutes + 45 minutes refrigeration   🕐 0 minutes   👤 5

INGREDIENTS

» 5 slices of bacon
» 3 large eggs, hard boiled
» ¼ cup shredded cheddar cheese
» ⅓ cup butter, softened
» 3 tablespoons mayonnaise
» Sea salt and pepper to taste

DIRECTIONS

1. Preheat the oven to 375°F. Line a baking sheet with parchment paper. Lay the bacon flat and bake for 10—15 minutes until golden brown. Reserve any bacon grease for later use.
2. Peel and quarter the hard boiled eggs.
3. Cut the butter into small pieces and mix with the eggs. Mash well with a fork.
4. Stir in the shredded cheese, mayonnaise and any leftover bacon grease. Season with salt and pepper. Mix well and place in the refrigerator for about 30—45 minutes, until firm.
5. Remove the egg mixture from the refrigerator and form into 5 balls.
6. Wrap each ball in a slice bacon and store in an airtight container until ready to serve.

- - - - - - - - - -

It's hard to argue that bacon isn't one of the tastiest foods in the world, but its reputation has been damaged over the last several decades. Believe it or not, bacon can be good for you, in moderation! It helps to stave off hunger, it raises your HDL, or "good" cholesterol levels, and it's a significant source of protein.

NUTRITION FACTS (PER SERVING)

Total Carbohydrates: 2g	Dietary Fiber: 0g	Net Carbs: 2g
Protein: 8g	Total Fat: 28g	Calories: 292

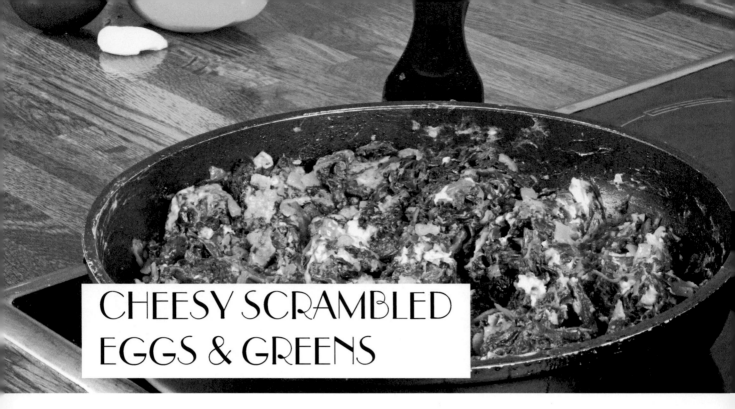

CHEESY SCRAMBLED EGGS & GREENS

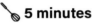 **5 minutes**   🕐 **10 minutes**   👤 **4**

INGREDIENTS

» 8 large eggs
» 6 cups kale, baby spinach, or Swiss Chard
» 1 cup shredded mozzarella cheese
» 2 tablespoons olive oil
» 2 tablespoons heavy cream
» Sea salt and pepper to taste
» Optional: for you meat lovers add some bacon and/or sausage while cooking the spinach, or for a non-meat option, top with half a sliced avocado.

DIRECTIONS

1. Crack the eggs into a medium bowl. Add the heavy cream to the eggs and season with salt and pepper. Whisk until well combined.
2. Roughly chop your greens.
3. Heat the olive oil in a large, non-stick pan over medium heat.
4. Add the baby spinach to the pan. Stir frequently, being careful not to burn. Once the spinach has wilted, reduce heat to low.
5. Add the egg mixture to the spinach and slowly stir until the eggs are almost set.
6. Add the cheddar cheese and stir until well combined.
7. Once the cheese has melted, divide onto four plates and serve!

Spinach is a low-calorie superfood loaded with nutrients that are important for skin and hair, bone health, and have strong anti-aging properties. And cooking it actually increases its health benefits!

NUTRITION FACTS (PER SERVING)

Total Carbohydrates: 6g	Dietary Fiber: 2g	Net Carbs: 4g
Protein: 16g	Total Fat: 19g	Calories: 251

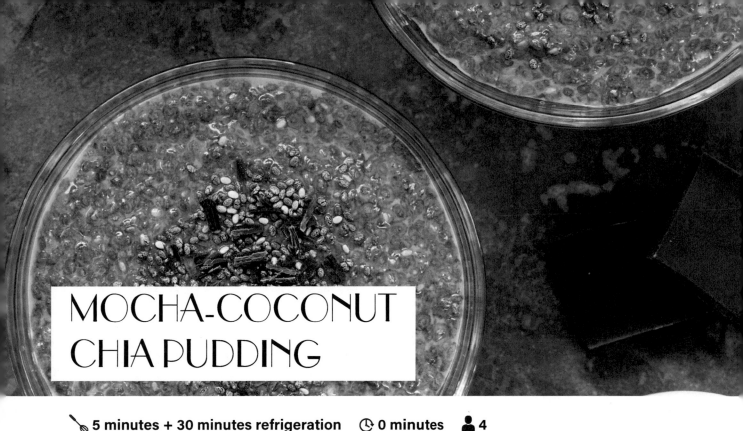

MOCHA-COCONUT CHIA PUDDING

🥄 **5 minutes + 30 minutes refrigeration**   ⏱ **0 minutes**   👤 **4**

INGREDIENTS

- » 4 tablespoons instant coffee
- » 2 tablespoons cocoa powder
- » ½ cup chia seeds
- » ½ cup coconut cream
- » 1 tablespoon vanilla extract
- » 2 tablespoons sugar substitute
- » 4 tablespoons cacao nibs
- » 2 cups water

DIRECTIONS

1. Prepare a strong cup of coffee by simmering the instant coffee with 2 cups of water for about 15 minutes, or until the liquid has reduced to about 1 cup.
2. Whisk the cocoa powder, coconut cream, vanilla extract, and sugar substitute into the coffee.
3. Stir in the chia seeds and cacao nibs. Mix well.
4. Divide into 4 small serving dishes and allow to set for at least 30 minutes.
5. Remove from refrigerator, garnish with a few additional cacao nibs, and serve!

Chia seeds are loaded with antioxidants whose job is to fight the production of free radicals, which damage the molecules in cells and contribute to diseases like cancer. Chia seeds take on a gelatinous texture once soaked in liquid, turning liquid into a rich and creamy pudding like magic.

NUTRITION FACTS (PER SERVING)

Total Carbohydrates: 14g	Dietary Fiber: 11g	Net Carbs: 3g
Protein: 7g	Total Fat: 21g	Calories: 257

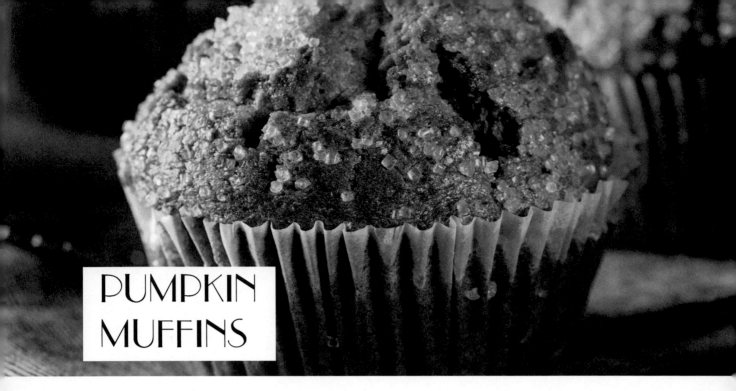

PUMPKIN MUFFINS

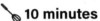 10 minutes   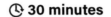 30 minutes   6

INGREDIENTS

- » ⅔ cup pumpkin puree
- » 1 ½ cups almond flour
- » 1 tablespoon pumpkin pie spice mix
- » ⅔ cup sugar substitute
- » 4 large eggs
- » 1 teaspoon baking powder

DIRECTIONS

1. Preheat oven to 300°F. Line a muffin pan with 6 paper liners.
2. In a large bowl, combine the almond flour, pumpkin pie spice, and sugar substitute. Mix well.
3. Add the pumpkin puree and eggs. Beat with an electric mixer until smooth.
4. Evenly divide the batter among the 6 paper liners and bake for 30—40 minutes, or until a toothpick inserted into the middle of a muffin comes out clean.
5. Remove from the oven and allow to cool on a wire rack.
6. Store in an airtight container until ready to serve.

The bright orange flesh of a pumpkin is loaded with fiber and key vitamins and minerals such as vitamin A, potassium, and iron. This delicious source of fiber is great for any time of year, not just for Thanksgiving and fall!

NUTRITION FACTS (PER SERVING)

Total Carbohydrates: 9g	Dietary Fiber: 6g	Net Carbs: 3g
Protein: 9g	Total Fat: 13g	Calories: 168

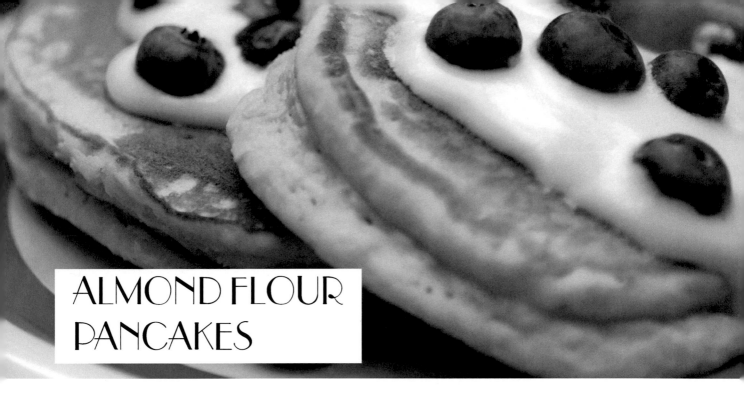

ALMOND FLOUR PANCAKES

 10 minutes   5—10 minutes   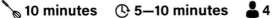 4

INGREDIENTS

» 1 cup almond flour
» 4 large eggs
» ¼ cup coconut oil, melted
» 1 teaspoon vanilla extract
» ¼ cup sugar substitute
» ½ teaspoon baking soda
» 1 teaspoon cream of tartar
» ¼ cup full-fat, plain yogurt
» ½ cup fresh blueberries (or berry of your choice)
» Additional coconut oil to grease the pan

DIRECTIONS

1. In a medium bowl, whisk the eggs until frothy.
2. In a separate bowl, mix together the almond flour, sugar substitute, baking soda, and cream of tartar until well combined.
3. Stir the vanilla extract and the melted coconut oil into the eggs.
4. Add the dry ingredients to the wet and mix well. Add a splash of water if the mixture seems too thick (it should be a bit thicker than regular pancake batter).
5. Grease a large skillet with about a teaspoon of coconut oil and spoon or ladle 2—3 small pancakes for every serving.
6. Cook on medium-low for about 5 minutes until the pancake starts to firm up. Flip and cook the other side for about a minute.
7. Remove from skillet, cover with foil to keep warm and repeat with remaining pancake batter.
8. Top each serving of pancakes with yogurt and berries.
9. Serve and enjoy!

Almond flour adds a wonderful flavor and texture to these pancakes. It's packed with vitamins and minerals, good for the heart, and each quarter cup contains 5 grams of protein.

NUTRITION FACTS (PER SERVING)

Total Carbohydrates: 9g	Dietary Fiber: 3g	Net Carbs: 6g
Protein: 12g	Total Fat: 33g	Calories: 368

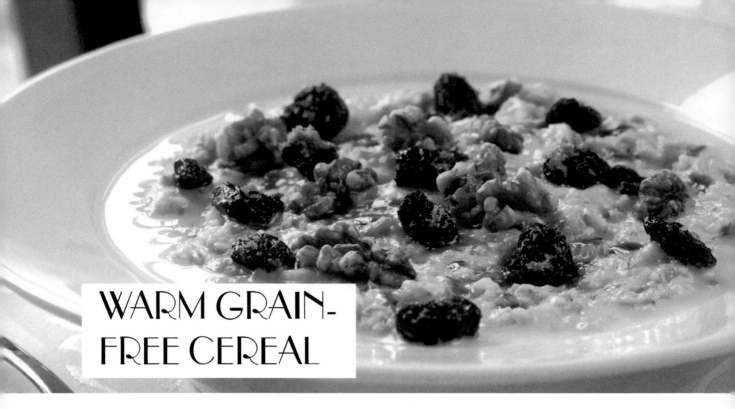

WARM GRAIN-FREE CEREAL

🥄 **5 minutes**   🕐 **8 minutes**   👤 **4**

INGREDIENTS

» 1 ⅓ cups of any combination of the following: crushed walnut pieces, sliced almonds, chopped macadamia nut pieces, toasted flaxseeds, hemp hearts, chia seeds, chopped cashews

» 6 tablespoons butter

» 1 cup unsweetened, shredded coconut

» 4 cups unsweetened almond milk

» Liquid stevia to taste (if desired)

» Pinch of salt

» If you have enough carb allowance left, try topping with fruit, raisins or, my favorite, blueberries.

DIRECTIONS

1. Preheat oven to 250°F. Toast the nuts and shredded coconut (keep separate from each other) until golden brown.

2. In a saucepan over medium heat, melt the butter.

3. Add the toasted nuts and a pinch of salt. Let cook for 1—2 minutes, stirring constantly. Add the toasted coconut and continue stirring.

4. Add the milk and liquid stevia, if using. Allow to cook for 5—7 minutes, until heated throughout.

5. Remove from heat, divide into 4 bowls and serve immediately.

Heart-healthy nuts take the place of grains in this warming breakfast. Nuts are a great source of unsaturated fats, which have been shown to help lower cholesterol levels.

NUTRITION FACTS (PER SERVING)

Total Carbohydrates: 10g	Dietary Fiber: 6g	Net Carbs: 4g
Protein: 9g	Total Fat: 62g	Calories: 603

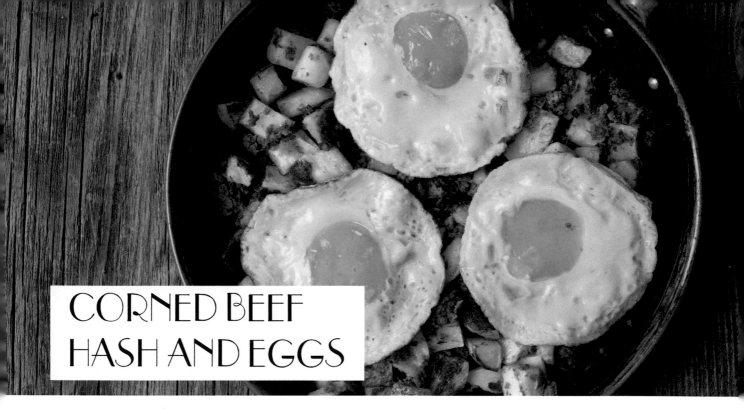

CORNED BEEF HASH AND EGGS

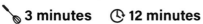 3 minutes   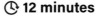 12 minutes   4

INGREDIENTS

» 2 cups cooked corned beef, chopped
» 4 large eggs
» 1 small yellow onion, diced
» 1 pound parsnips, peeled and diced
» 2 cloves garlic, minced
» ½ cup beef or chicken broth
» 2 tablespoons olive oil
» Sea salt and pepper to taste

DIRECTIONS

1. Heat olive oil in a large skillet over medium high heat.
2. Add the onions and garlic and sautè for 1—2 minutes, until translucent.
3. Add the parsnips and cook for another 5 minutes.
4. Reduce heat to medium-low, pour in the beef broth, cover and cook for 5 minutes, until the parsnips are tender and the liquid has been absorbed.
5. Add the chopped corned beef and stir until well combined.
6. Carefully crack the eggs on top of the hash, season with salt and pepper, cover, and continue cooking for 5—7 minutes, or until eggs are cooked to your desired level of doneness.
7. Serve immediately.

Parsnips are a root vegetable closely related to the carrot. They contain a wide variety of minerals and nutrients, including dietary fiber, folate, potassium, and vitamin C.

NUTRITION FACTS (PER SERVING)

Total Carbohydrates: 14g	Dietary Fiber: 6g	Net Carbs: 8g
Protein: 23g	Total Fat: 26g	Calories: 416

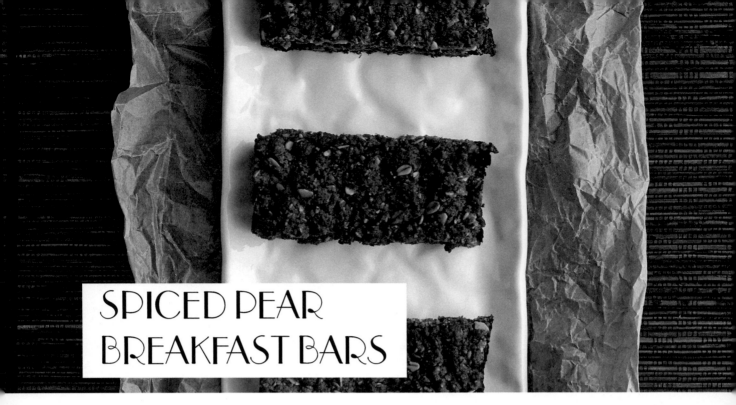

SPICED PEAR BREAKFAST BARS

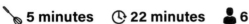

🥄 **5 minutes**   🕐 **22 minutes**   👤 **6**

INGREDIENTS

- » 1 large pear, cored and peeled
- » 3 large eggs
- » 2 tablespoons coconut oil
- » 2 tablespoons maple syrup
- » ¼ cup coconut flour
- » 1 teaspoon cinnamon
- » ½ teaspoon nutmeg
- » ¼ teaspoon cloves
- » ½ teaspoon baking soda
- » ¼ teaspoon salt

DIRECTIONS

1. Preheat oven to 350°F. Prepare an 8x8 baking dish with non-stick spray.
2. In a food processor, pulse the apple until pureed. Add the eggs, maple syrup, and coconut oil. Blend until well combined.
3. Add the salt, baking soda, cinnamon, nutmeg, cloves, and coconut flour. Mix until just combined.
4. Pour the batter into the prepared pan. Sprinkle with additional cinnamon, if desired.
5. Bake for 22—25 minutes, or until a toothpick inserted comes out clean.
6. Allow to cool on a wire rack. Cut into 6 squares. Wrap individual pieces in plastic wrap and store in the freezer for a quick breakfast throughout the week!

Cinnamon is not only delicious, but it's one of the healthiest spices on the planet! It can help lower blood sugar levels and reduce heart disease risk factors. It's also loaded with powerful antioxidants.

NUTRITION FACTS (PER SERVING)

Total Carbohydrates: 10g	Dietary Fiber: 1g	Net Carbs: 9g
Protein: 4g	Total Fat: 9g	Calories: 127

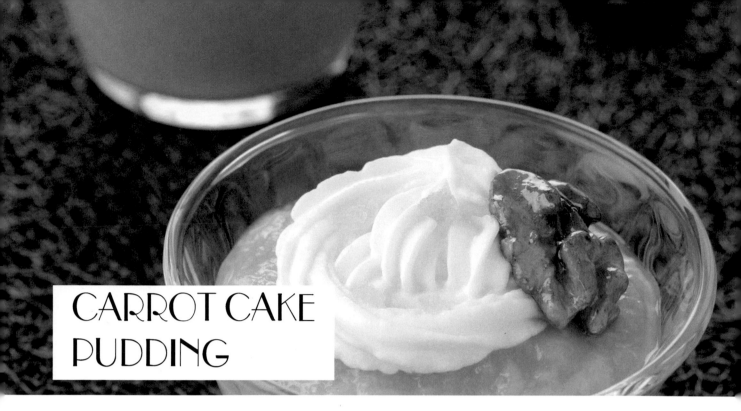

CARROT CAKE PUDDING

 5 minutes   **20 minutes**   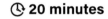 **4**

INGREDIENTS

» 2 cups peeled and chopped carrots
» 2 tablespoons coconut cream
» 2 tablespoons almond butter
» 1 teaspoon vanilla extract
» ½ teaspoon cinnamon
» ½ teaspoon nutmeg
» ¼ teaspoon cloves
» Pinch of sea salt
» Optional garnish: Heavy cream, whipped to stiff peaks and/or toasted nuts

DIRECTIONS

1. Place the carrots in a medium saucepan and cover with water.
2. Cook over medium-high heat for 10—15 minutes, until fork tender.
3. Drain the carrots and place in a food processor.
4. Add the rest of the ingredients to the food processor and puree until smooth and creamy.
5. Divide into 4 serving dishes, garnish with whipped cream if desired, and enjoy! Sometimes, I also like to top with nuts; the nutty flavor complements the pudding.
6. Store leftovers in an airtight container in the fridge.

Carrots are a powerhouse of a vegetable. Just one serving contains 11% of your daily vitamin A needs. They also contain high amounts of beta-carotene, which is important for vision, immunity, and overall health.

NUTRITION FACTS (PER SERVING)

Total Carbohydrates: 11g	Dietary Fiber: 4g	Net Carbs: 7g
Protein: 3g	Total Fat: 7g	Calories: 108

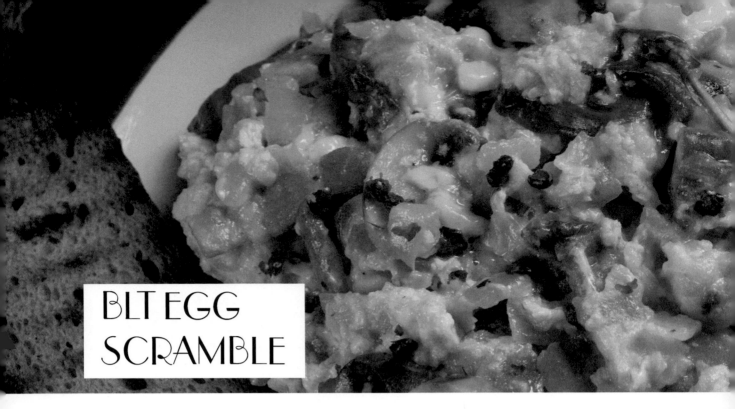

BLT EGG SCRAMBLE

🥄 5 minutes   🕐 15 minutes   👤 4

INGREDIENTS

- » 4 slices bacon, cooked and chopped
- » 2 cups baby spinach
- » ½ cup diced tomatoes
- » ½ cup sliced mushrooms
- » 1 avocado, diced
- » 6 large eggs
- » 2 tablespoons sour cream
- » 1 tablespoon coconut oil
- » Sea salt and pepper to taste
- » Optional: 1 slice of low-carb bread

DIRECTIONS

1. Lightly beat the eggs and sour cream together in a bowl.
2. Heat the coconut oil in a large skillet over medium heat.
3. Cook the egg mixture for about 5—7 minutes, stirring constantly.
4. Gently fold in the bacon, tomatoes, avocado, and spinach.
5. Continue cooking for another 2—3 minutes, until the spinach begins to wilt.
6. Remove from heat, season with salt and pepper, and enjoy! Serve with a slice of low-carb toast, if you have room in your daily carb allowance.

Once touted as being not so heart healthy, eggs have since been recognized to have plenty of nutritional benefits. And eating the whole egg is vital to reaping all of its benefits.

NUTRITION FACTS (PER SERVING)

Total Carbohydrates: 10g	Dietary Fiber: 5g	Net Carbs: 5g
Protein: 21g	Total Fat: 33g	Calories: 412

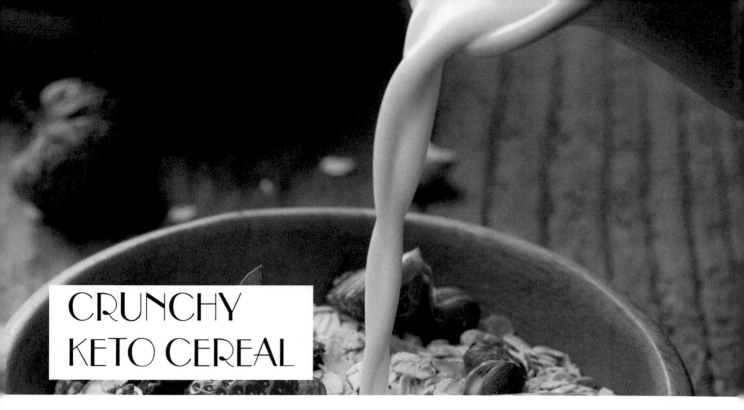

CRUNCHY KETO CEREAL

🥄 **5 minutes**   🕐 **8 minutes**   👤 **4**

INGREDIENTS

» 2 cups unsweetened coconut flakes
» 1 cup sliced almonds
» ½ cup sunflower seeds
» ¼ cup walnuts
» 4 tablespoons coconut oil
» 2 tablespoons cinnamon
» 4 tablespoons sugar substitute
» Unsweetened almond or coconut milk for serving
» 1 cup fresh strawberries

DIRECTIONS

1. Preheat oven to 350°F.
2. Place the coconut flakes, sliced almonds, sunflower seeds, and walnuts in a large bowl.
3. In a small saucepan over medium heat, combine the coconut oil, cinnamon, and sugar substitute. Stir until well combined and heat through.
4. Pour the mixture over the coconut flakes and nuts and toss to coat.
5. Spread the coconut onto a rimmed baking sheet. Bake for 5—8 minutes, stirring every couple of minutes to prevent from burning.
6. Allow to cool and serve with unsweetened milk of your choice and topped with fresh berries.

- - - - - - - -

Considered one of the most treasured foods of all time, the coconut delivers superb health benefits, including blood sugar stabilization, improved digestion, and lower cholesterol.

NUTRITION FACTS (PER SERVING)

| Total Carbohydrates: 17g | Dietary Fiber: 9g | Net Carbs: 8g |
| Protein: 10g | Total Fat: 48g | Calories: 510 |

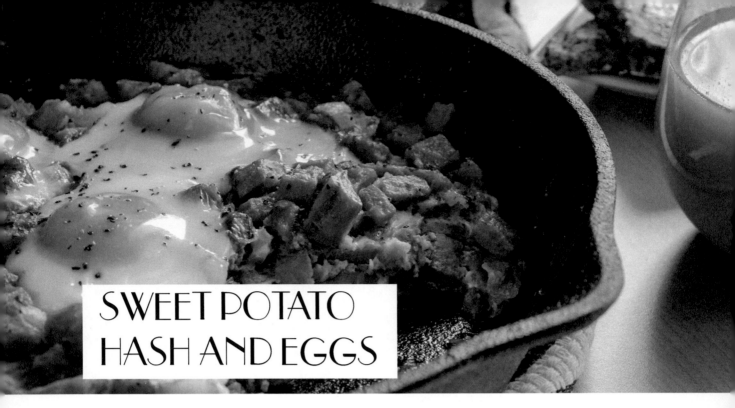

SWEET POTATO HASH AND EGGS

🥄 5 minutes   🕐 10 minutes   👤 4

INGREDIENTS

» 2 large sweet potatoes
» 4 large eggs
» ½ yellow onion, diced
» 3 cloves garlic, minced
» 2 tablespoons coconut oil
» Sea salt and pepper to taste

DIRECTIONS

1. Shred your sweet potatoes using a food processor. Alternatively, you can grate them using the large holes on a cheese grater.
2. Heat the coconut oil in a large skillet over medium heat. Once hot, add the sweet potato, onions, and garlic to the pan. Cook, stirring every couple of minutes, for about 10—12 minutes.
3. Set your oven to broil on high.
4. Evenly spread the sweet potato mixture across the skillet and create 4 wells with the back of a spoon.
5. Crack the eggs into the wells and place under the broiler.
6. Cook for 2—3 minutes, until the egg whites are opaque.
7. Remove from broiler and season with salt and pepper.
8. Allow to rest for about 5 minutes before serving.

Sweet potatoes are a great source of vitamin A, which supports the immune system. Just one serving contains more than 10of the daily recommended dose of vitamin A.

NUTRITION FACTS (PER SERVING)

Total Carbohydrates: 16g	Dietary Fiber: 4g	Net Carbs: 12g
Protein: 7g	Total Fat: 11g	Calories: 216

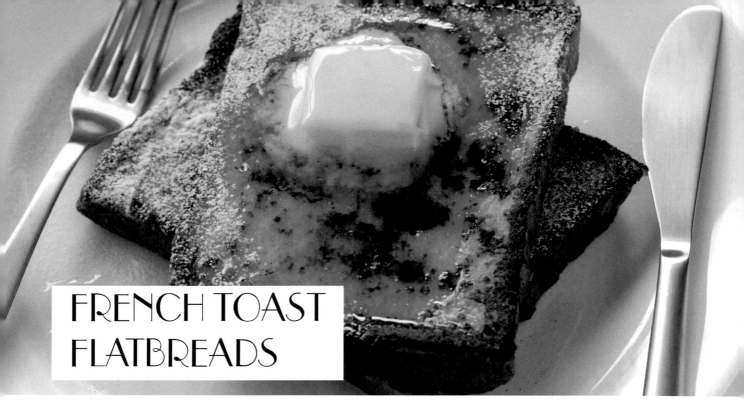

FRENCH TOAST FLATBREADS

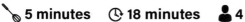 **5 minutes**   **18 minutes**   **4**

INGREDIENTS

- » ¼ cup arrowroot flour
- » ¼ cup coconut flour
- » ¼ cup canned coconut milk
- » ¼ cup maple syrup
- » 6 eggs, separated
- » 2 teaspoons cinnamon
- » ½ teaspoon nutmeg
- » ½ teaspoon vanilla extract

DIRECTIONS

1. Preheat oven to 350°F. Prepare an 8x8 baking dish with non-stick spray.
2. Using a stand mixer or hand mixer, beat the egg whites until stiff peaks form.
3. In a small bowl, mix the egg yolks, maple syrup, cinnamon, nutmeg, coconut milk, and vanilla extract until well combined.
4. Gently pour the yolk mixture into the egg whites and stir until combined.
5. Slowly fold in the arrowroot flour and coconut flour until just combined.
6. Pour into the prepared baking dish and bake for 18 minutes, until golden brown and spongy to the touch.
7. Slice into squares and enjoy warm or wrap and refrigerate for later.
8. If you have more time, serve it as part of a traditional brunch, alongside eggs, bacon, sausages etc.

Arrowroot powder is similar to cornstarch but much lower in carbs. It can be used to thicken soups and sauces, or as a flour substitute, as used in this recipe.

NUTRITION FACTS (PER SERVING)

Total Carbohydrates: 11g	Dietary Fiber: 2g	Net Carbs: 9g
Protein: 7g	Total Fat: 8g	Calories: 138

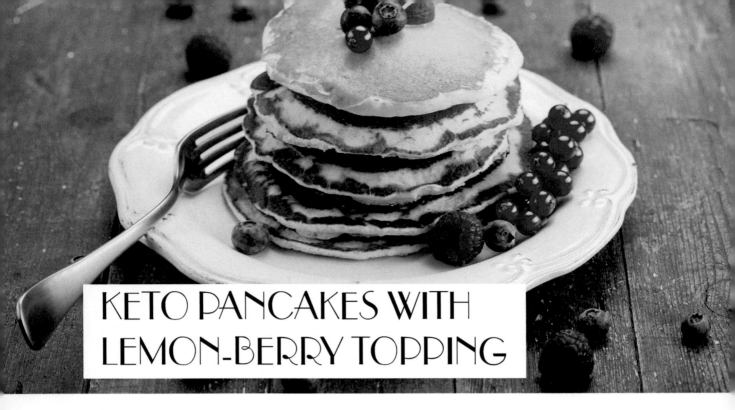

KETO PANCAKES WITH LEMON-BERRY TOPPING

 5 minutes **8 minutes** **4**

INGREDIENTS

»   3 eggs, whisked
»   ½ cup coconut flour
»   ½ cup tapioca flour
»   ⅔ cup unsweetened almond milk
»   1 tablespoon maple syrup
»   1 teaspoon vanilla extract
»   ½ teaspoon baking powder
»   ½ teaspoon baking soda
»   Pinch of salt
»   Coconut oil for greasing the pan

Topping:

»   ½ cup raspberries
»   ½ cup blueberries
»   Juice of one lemon
»   1 tablespoon honey

DIRECTIONS

1. In a saucepan over medium heat, simmer the topping ingredients, stirring frequently.
2. For the pancakes: whisk together the eggs, almond milk, honey, and vanilla extract.
3. Slowly whisk in the coconut flour, tapioca flour, baking powder, and baking soda until well combined.
4. Grease a large skillet with coconut oil and place over medium heat. Once the pan is hot, ladle the pancake mixture into the pan.
5. Place about a tablespoon of the raspberry mixture into the pancake and swirl. Once bubbles begin to surface, carefully flip and cook for 2—3 minutes.
6. Remove from the pan and repeat with the remaining pancake mixture.
7. Serve with the remaining raspberry and blueberry mixture and enjoy!

Raspberries contain antioxidants such as Vitamin C, quercetin, and gallic acid which help prevent circulatory disease and age-related decline. They are also high in ellagic acid which has been shown to have anti-inflammatory properties.

NUTRITION FACTS (PER SERVING)

Total Carbohydrates: 20g	Dietary Fiber: 8g	Net Carbs: 12g
Protein: 8g	Total Fat: 10g	Calories: 201

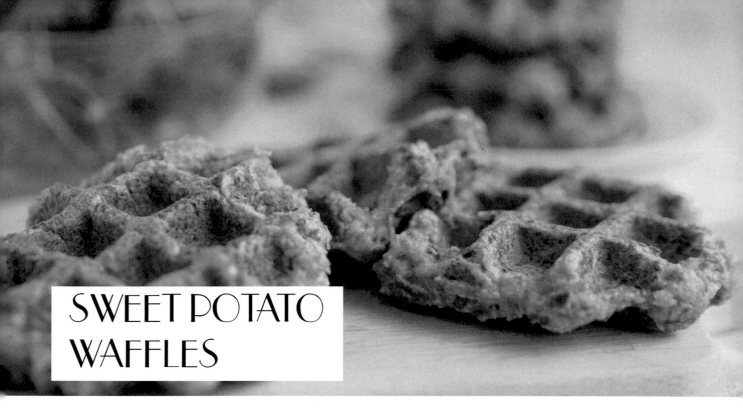

SWEET POTATO WAFFLES

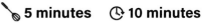 5 minutes   10 minutes   👤 4

INGREDIENTS

» 3 medium sweet potatoes, peeled and grated
» 4 large eggs, lightly beaten
» 3 tablespoons coconut oil, melted
» 3 tablespoons coconut flour
» 1 teaspoon cinnamon
» ½ teaspoon nutmeg
» Optional topping: sour cream

DIRECTIONS

1. Combine all of the ingredients, except the sour cream, in a large bowl. Mix until well combined.
2. Cook in batches in your waffle maker. Keep the waffles on the thinner side to ensure the sweet potatoes cook through.
3. Remove from the waffle maker and top with sour cream, if desired.

Don't have a waffle maker? These can easily be turned into pancakes. Just heat some oil in a large skillet over medium-high heat and cook as you would regular pancakes.

NUTRITION FACTS (PER SERVING)

Total Carbohydrates: 18g	Dietary Fiber: 4g	Net Carbs: 14g
Protein: 8g	Total Fat: 17g	Calories: 265

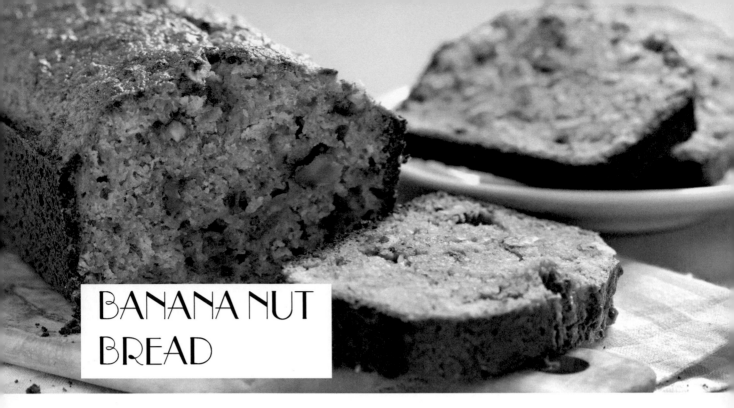

BANANA NUT BREAD

🥄 **10 minutes**   🕐 **45 minutes**   👤 **6**

INGREDIENTS

» 3 very ripe bananas, mashed
» 3 large eggs
» ½ cup almond butter
» 3 tablespoons coconut oil
» ¼ cup walnuts
» ½ cup coconut flour
» 1 tablespoon cinnamon
» 1 teaspoon baking soda
» 1 teaspoon baking powder
» 1 teaspoon vanilla extract
» Pinch of sea salt

DIRECTIONS

1. Preheat oven to 350°F. Prepare a 9x5 inch loaf pan with non-stick spray.
2. Combine the mashed bananas, eggs, almond butter, and coconut oil in a blender or food processor. Blend until smooth and creamy.
3. Add the coconut flour, cinnamon, baking soda, baking powder, and vanilla extract and blend until well combined.
4. Pour the batter into your prepared loaf pan and sprinkle with the walnuts. Bake for 45—55 minutes, until a toothpick inserted into the center comes out clean.
5. Allow to cool on a wire rack. Slice and serve!

Bananas are one of the most widely consumed fruits in the world, and for good reason. The fiber, potassium, vitamin C and B6 content in bananas all help to support heart health.

NUTRITION FACTS (PER SERVING)

Total Carbohydrates: 16g	Dietary Fiber: 4g	Net Carbs: 12g
Protein: 11g	Total Fat: 28g	Calories: 353

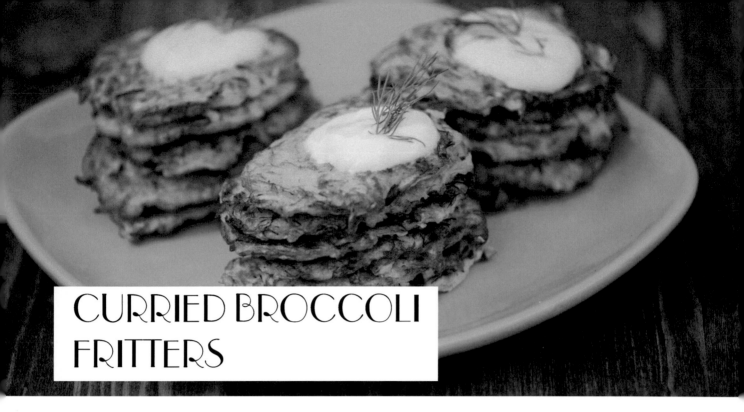

CURRIED BROCCOLI FRITTERS

 5 minutes   🕐 **10 minutes**   👤 **4**

INGREDIENTS

» 4 cups roasted or steamed broccoli florets (measure after cooking)
» 1 cup shredded carrots
» 1 tablespoon curry powder
» 1 tablespoon coconut flour or almond flour
» 4 eggs
» Sea salt and pepper to taste
» Coconut oil for the pan
» Optional toppings: sour cream, whipped heavy cream, coconut cream

DIRECTIONS

1. In a food processor, pulse the broccoli florets until finely ground.
2. Add the shredded carrots, egg, curry powder, and coconut flour. Season with salt and pepper. Process to combine.
3. The batter should be thick enough to hold its shape in the skillet. If it seems too thin, add a bit more coconut flour, about a teaspoon at a time.
4. Heat about a tablespoon of coconut oil in a large skillet over medium-high heat.
5. Drop the batter into the hot pan, about 2 tablespoons for each fritter.
6. Cook until golden brown on each side. Repeat with the remaining batter.

Broccoli has a strong, positive impact on our body's detoxification system, ridding the body of unwanted contaminates while helping to neutralize PH levels.

NUTRITION FACTS (PER SERVING)

Total Carbohydrates: 10g	Dietary Fiber: 3g	Net Carbs: 7g
Protein: 9g	Total Fat: 14g	Calories: 185

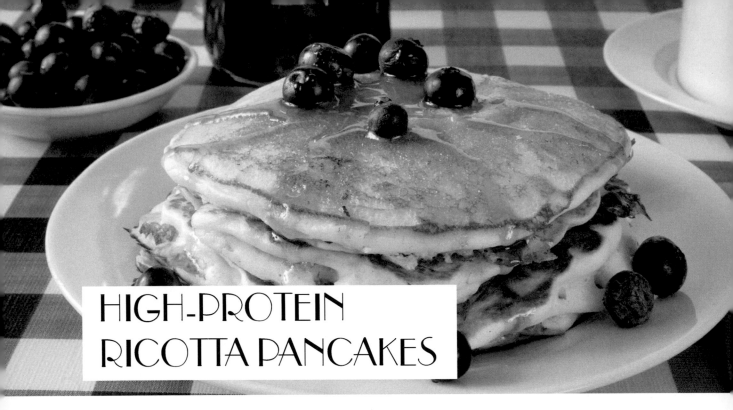

HIGH-PROTEIN RICOTTA PANCAKES

🥄 **5 minutes**   🕐 **10 minutes**   👤 **4**

INGREDIENTS

» 8 eggs
» ⅔ cup flax meal
» 1 ½ cups ricotta cheese
» 1 tablespoon honey
» 2 teaspoons baking powder
» ½ teaspoon salt
» 1 cup fresh blueberries for topping

DIRECTIONS

1. Combine the flax meal, baking powder and salt in a large bowl. Add the eggs to the dry ingredients one by one, whisking after each egg.

2. Whisk in the ricotta cheese and honey and mix until smooth and creamy. Alternatively, put the above ingredients into a blender and blend on high to achieve the same results.

3. Spray a griddle or non-stick skillet with non-stick cooking spray and set over medium-high heat.

4. Once the skillet is hot, use a large spoon or preferably a ladle (this is the perfect size for pancake batter) to pour the pancake batter into the skillet.

5. Allow the pancake to cook for about 2 minutes before flipping it over with a spatula. Cook the other side for about 2 minutes. Adjust the timing accordingly if you would prefer your pancakes more or less browned.

6. Repeat with the remaining batter.

- - - - - - - - - - - - - - - - - -

Top the pancakes with fresh blueberries and serve with butter, low-carb syrup, crème fraiche, or any combination of these options!

NUTRITION FACTS (PER SERVING)

Total Carbohydrates: 22g	Dietary Fiber: 12g	Net Carbs: 10g
Protein: 30g	Total Fat: 30g	Calories: 451

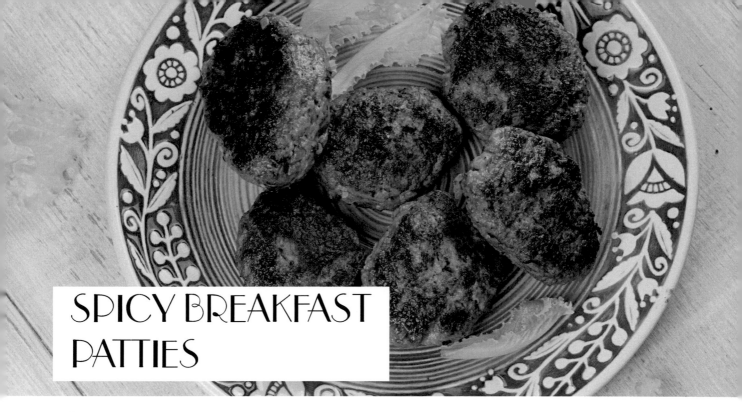

SPICY BREAKFAST PATTIES

🥄 10 minutes   🕐 10 minutes   👤 4

INGREDIENTS

» 1 pound ground pork
» 1 teaspoon smoked paprika
» 1 teaspoon garlic powder
» 1 teaspoon fennel seed
» ½ teaspoon crushed red pepper
» ½ teaspoon thyme
» ½ teaspoon cayenne pepper
» ¼ teaspoon sea salt
» ¼ teaspoon black pepper
» 2 tablespoons coconut oil

DIRECTIONS

1. Combine the pork with all of the spices in a large mixing bowl. Mix well with hands, until the spices are fully incorporated.
2. Form the pork mixture into 8 patties.
3. Heat 1 tablespoon of the coconut oil in a large skillet over medium-high heat.
4. Cook the patties for about 8—10 minutes, turning occasionally.
5. Repeat with the remaining patties and coconut oil.
6. Wonderful when served alongside a scrambled or fried egg.

Lean pork is an abundant source of protein and is loaded with minerals like magnesium and calcium which are known to strengthen the immune system.

NUTRITION FACTS (PER SERVING)

Total Carbohydrates: 0g	Dietary Fiber: 0g	Net Carbs: 0g
Protein: 30g	Total Fat: 11g	Calories: 221

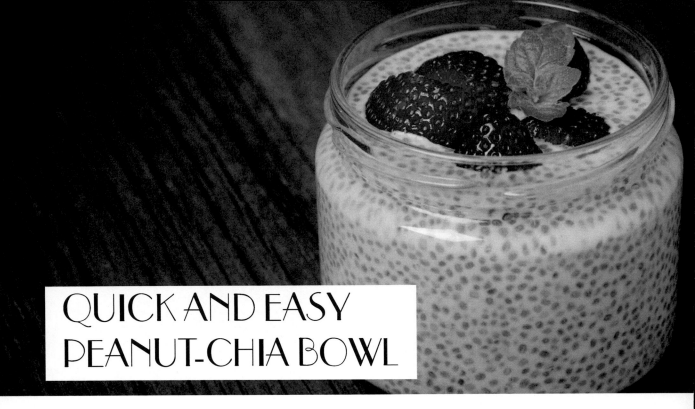

QUICK AND EASY PEANUT-CHIA BOWL

🥄 2 minutes   🕐 3 minutes   👤 4

INGREDIENTS

- » ⅓ cup chia seeds
- » ⅔ cup peanut flour
- » 2 cup unsweetened almond milk
- » 4 scoops vanilla protein powder
- » 1 tablespoon ground cinnamon
- » ¼ cup ground flaxseeds
- » 1 cup water

Suggested toppings

- » Toasted almonds
- » Hemp hearts
- » Toasted coconut
- » Almond butter
- » Favorite fruit

DIRECTIONS

1. For the most flavor, it is best to prepare this the night before to allow the ingredients to marinate. The night before, combine the almond milk and water together in one bowl. Combine all dry ingredients (except the ground flaxseeds) in another. Make a well in the dry ingredients and pour the liquid, a little at a time, into the dry ingredients while continuously whisking. Whisk until well combined. Cover the bowl and refrigerate overnight.

2. The next day, place the mixture in a saucepan over medium heat. Bring the mixture to a simmer, stirring frequently. The thickness should not be too runny, but not solid either. This can be to your personal preference.

3. Stir in the flaxseeds once you are ready to serve. Divide evenly among 4 bowls and add your favorite toppings.

NUTRITION FACTS (PER SERVING)

Total Carbohydrates: 13g	Dietary Fiber: 7g	Net Carbs: 6g
Protein: 30g	Total Fat: 20g	Calories: 326

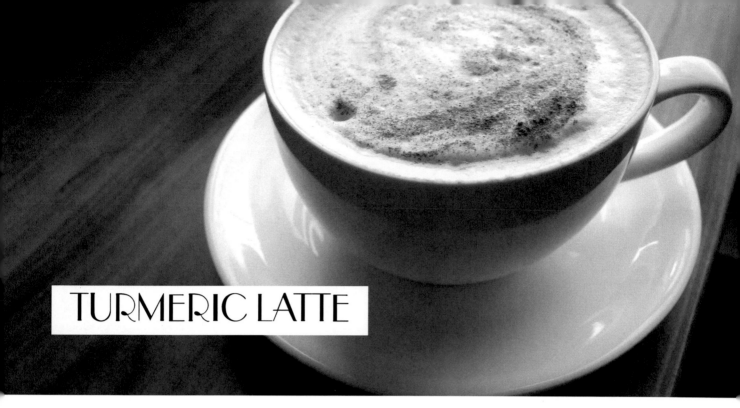

TURMERIC LATTE

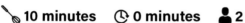 **10 minutes**   **0 minutes**   **2**

INGREDIENTS

- » 16 ounces strongly brewed coffee
- » 1 teaspoon turmeric
- » ½ teaspoon cinnamon
- » 2 tablespoons grass-fed butter
- » 1 teaspoon coconut oil
- » Optional: 2 teaspoons honey

DIRECTIONS

1. Brew the coffee with the cinnamon and turmeric. (A French press works great, but any method of brewing coffee will work — just add the spices to the coffee grounds.)
2. Pour the hot coffee into a high speed blender with the butter and coconut oil. Blend until frothy.
3. Divide between 2 large mugs and enjoy!

Turmeric is a powerful spice that has been used in Chinese and Indian medicine for centuries. It has anti-inflammatory properties and adds a warm, peppery flavor.

NUTRITION FACTS (PER SERVING)

Total Carbohydrates: 6g	Dietary Fiber: 0g	Net Carbs: 6g
Protein: 0g	Total Fat: 14g	Calories: 145

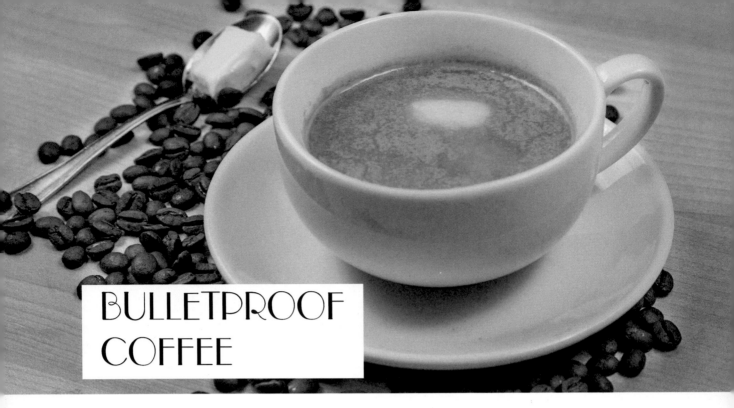

BULLETPROOF COFFEE

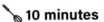 **10 minutes**   🕐 **0 minutes**   👤 **2**

INGREDIENTS

- » 16 ounces strongly brewed coffee
- » 2 tablespoons grass-fed butter
- » 2 tablespoons coconut oil
- » 2 tablespoons heavy cream
- » 1 teaspoon vanilla extract

DIRECTIONS

1. Brew the coffee as you normally would.
2. Pour the hot coffee into a high speed blender with the butter, coconut oil, heavy cream, and vanilla extract. Blend until frothy.
3. Pour into 2 large mugs and enjoy!

Consuming healthy fats such as grass-fed butter and coconut oil has been shown to lead to greater amounts of energy and more effective weight loss.

NUTRITION FACTS (PER SERVING)

Total Carbohydrates: 0g	Dietary Fiber: 0g	Net Carbs: 0g
Protein: 1g	Total Fat: 31g	Calories: 273

WEEKEND / BRUNCH RECIPES

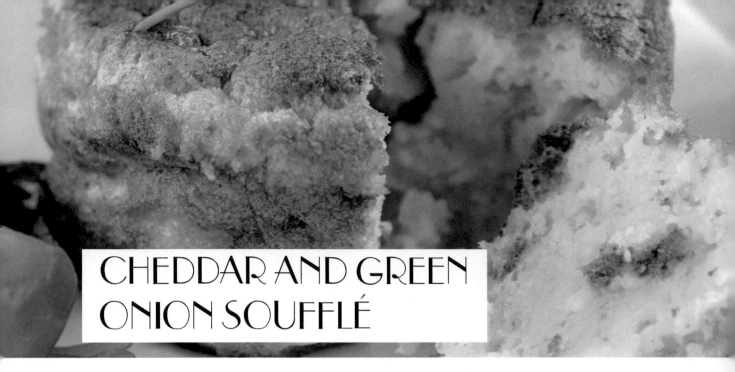

CHEDDAR AND GREEN ONION SOUFFLÉ

 10 minutes   25 minutes   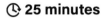 4

INGREDIENTS

» 6 large eggs, separated
» 2 cups shredded cheddar cheese
» 1 bunch green onions, thinly sliced
» ¾ cup heavy cream
» ½ cup almond flour
» 1 teaspoon ground mustard
» ½ teaspoon xanthan gum
» ¼ teaspoon cayenne pepper
» ¼ teaspoon cream of tartar
» Sea salt and pepper to taste

DIRECTIONS

1. Preheat the oven to 350°F. Grease 4 (6—8 ounce) ramekins and place on a baking sheet.
2. In a large bowl, whisk together the almond flour, mustard, xanthan gum, cayenne, salt, and pepper.
3. Slowly whisk in the heavy cream until well combined. Continue whisking and add the cheese, green onions, and egg yolks until fully incorporated.
4. In a large, clean bowl, beat the egg whites with the cream of tartar until stiff peaks form.
5. Carefully fold the egg whites into the yolk mixture until just combined.
6. Divide the mixture evenly among the prepared ramekins and carefully place the baking sheet into the oven. Bake for about 20—25 minutes or until the soufflès have risen about an inch or two above the rim and are golden brown.
7. Serve immediately.

- - - - - - - - - - - - - -
Baking a soufflè is easier than you think. The key is to handle the egg whites with care and not overmix them. The addition of xanthan gum in this recipe acts a stabilizer to the eggs, helping prevent them from deflating.

NUTRITION FACTS (PER SERVING)

Total Carbohydrates: 4g	Dietary Fiber: 2g	Net Carbs: 2g
Protein: 25g	Total Fat: 40g	Calories: 468

32

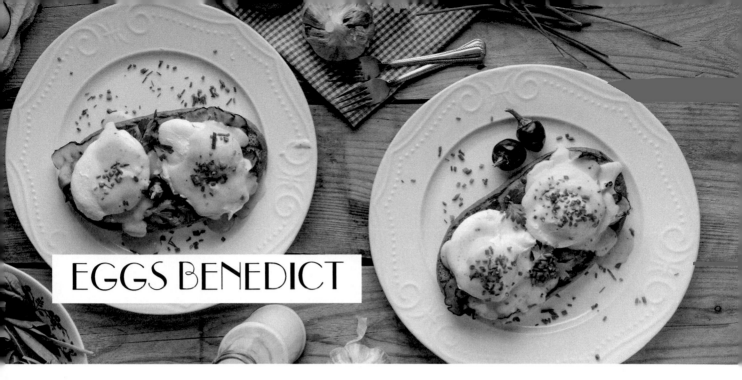

EGGS BENEDICT

🥄 **10 minutes**   🕐 **30 minutes**   👤 **4**

INGREDIENTS

» 8 ham or prosciutto slices
» 8 large eggs

Protein Bun
» 3 eggs, separated
» ¼ cup unflavored protein powder
» 2 tablespoons coconut flour

Hollandaise Sauce
» 3 egg yolks
» ¼ cup lemon juice
» 1 tablespoon Dijon mustard
» ½ cup butter, melted
» Sea salt and pepper to taste

DIRECTIONS

1. To make the buns: Preheat oven to 325°F.
2. Separate the eggs (reserve the egg yolks) and whip the egg whites until stiff peaks form.
3. Gently mix in the protein powder and coconut flour.
4. Grease a baking sheet and evenly divide the mixture into 4 mounds, about the size of a hamburger bun, onto the sheet. Bake for 15—20 minutes or until golden brown.
5. Allow to cool completely before slicing in half lengthwise.
6. To prepare the hollandaise sauce: Place the reserved egg yolks, lemon juice, and Dijon mustard in the top of a double boiler set over simmering water. Whisk to blend.
7. Whisking constantly, add the melted butter in a slow, steady stream. Cook the sauce, whisking constantly, until thickened. Season with salt and pepper and remove from heat.
8. To assemble: Slice a bun in half, plate, and top each half with a slice of ham or prosciutto. Top each half with poached egg and 2—3 tablespoons hollandaise sauce. Serve immediately.

Egg poaching tip: Add a few tablespoons of vinegar to gently simmering water — it will help hold the egg whites together. 4 minutes will give you firm egg whites with a soft yolk. Leave it in a minute longer and you'll have a yolk that's custardy and soft.

NUTRITION FACTS (PER SERVING)

Total Carbohydrates: 5g	Dietary Fiber: 1g	Net Carbs: 4g
Protein: 38g	Total Fat: 44g	Calories: 568

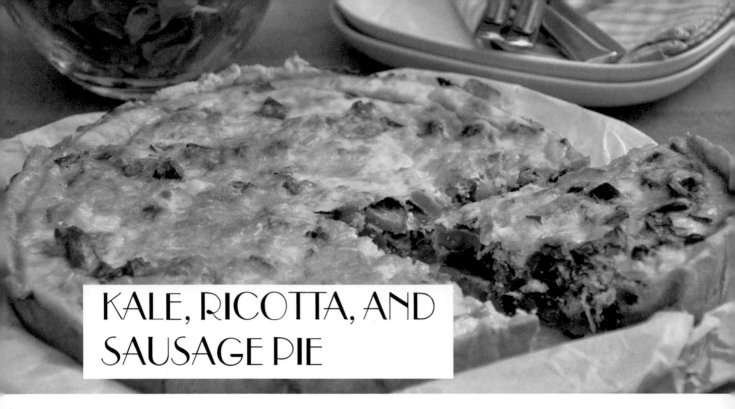

KALE, RICOTTA, AND SAUSAGE PIE

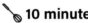 **10 minutes**   ⏱ **30—35 minutes**   👤 **6**

INGREDIENTS

- » 6 cups kale, chopped
- » 1 ½ cups ricotta cheese
- » 1 pound breakfast sausage
- » 4 eggs
- » 1 cup shredded cheddar cheese
- » ½ yellow onion, diced
- » 3 cloves garlic, minced
- » 2 tablespoons olive oil
- » Sea salt and pepper to taste

DIRECTIONS

1. Preheat oven to 350°F.
2. Heat the olive oil in a large skillet and add the onions and garlic. Cook until softened. Add the kale and cook for about 5 minutes, until wilted. Season with salt and pepper and remove from heat.
3. Beat the eggs in a large bowl. Add the ricotta and shredded cheddar. Stir in the sautéed kale.
4. Roll out the breakfast sausage and press it into a 9-inch pie pan, making sure to go up the sides of the pan.
5. Pour in the filling and place on a baking sheet to catch any drippings from the sausage. Bake for 30—35 minutes, until the eggs are set.
6. Allow to rest for 5—10 minutes, slice into 6 pieces and serve!

This savory breakfast pie is easy to throw together, packed with protein, and extremely versatile. Try swapping out the kale for spinach or Swiss chard or the cheddar cheese for mozzarella.

NUTRITION FACTS (PER SERVING)

Total Carbohydrates: 11g	Dietary Fiber: 1g	Net Carbs: 10g
Protein: 32g	Total Fat: 40g	Calories: 533

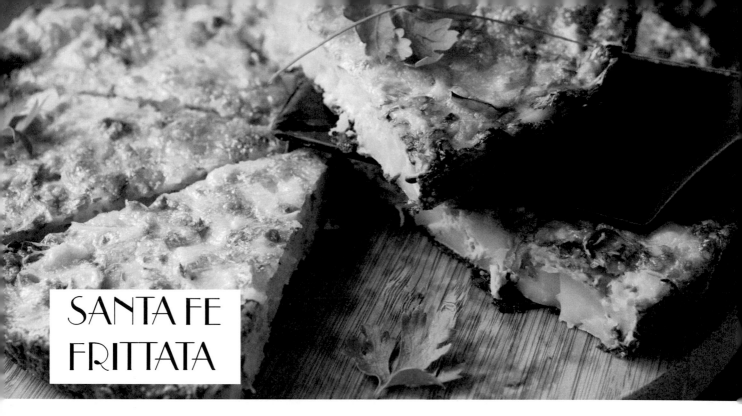

SANTA FE FRITTATA

🥄 10 minutes   🕐 30 minutes   👤 6

INGREDIENTS

- » 8 ounces diced ham
- » 2 bell peppers, any color, diced
- » ½ red onion, diced
- » 8-10 cherry tomatoes, quartered
- » ½ cup fresh cilantro, chopped
- » ⅔ cup shredded pepper jack cheese
- » 10 large eggs
- » 2 egg whites
- » ½ cup milk
- » Sea salt and pepper to taste
- » Optional garnishes: Diced green onions, salsa, sour cream

DIRECTIONS

1. Preheat oven to 350°F. Grease a 9-inch glass pie pan.
2. Brown the ham in a large skillet until golden brown. Remove from pan and set aside.
3. Using the same skillet, cook the peppers, onion and cherry tomatoes until softened.
4. In a large bowl, whisk together the eggs, egg whites and milk.
5. Evenly sprinkle the sausage and veggies into the prepared pie pan. Top with the chopped cilantro. Pour the egg mixture on top and season with salt and pepper.
6. Top with the shredded cheese and bake for 25—30 minutes, or until set.
7. Allow to cool for 5—10 minutes and slice into 6 servings.
8. Top with optional garnishes and enjoy!

To maximize the benefit of a vegetable rich diet, it's important to eat a variety of colors and this veggie packed frittata does just that. The peppers, onion, and cherry tomatoes provide a wide range of vitamin and nutrients as well as a healthy dose of fiber.

NUTRITION FACTS (PER SERVING)

Total Carbohydrates: 5g	Dietary Fiber: 1g	Net Carbs: 4g
Protein: 21g	Total Fat: 16g	Calories: 245

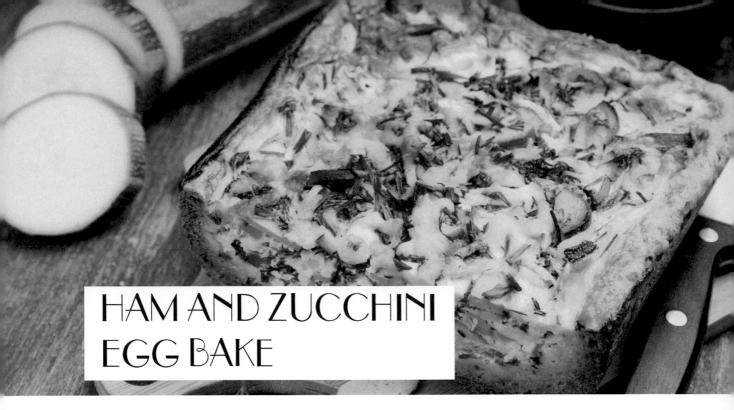

HAM AND ZUCCHINI EGG BAKE

 5 minutes   **20—25 minutes**   **6**

INGREDIENTS

- » 4 small zucchini, cut into ½-inch thick rounds
- » 6 slices ham or Canadian bacon
- » ½ cup grated Asiago cheese
- » 6 large eggs
- » 1 small bunch parsley, chopped
- » Sea salt and pepper to taste

DIRECTIONS

1. Preheat oven to 350°F. Prepare an 8x8 baking dish with non-stick spray.
2. Cut the ham slices in half, then cut each half lengthwise into ¼" thick strips.
3. Cook the ham strips in a large skillet over medium heat for about 3 minutes, until golden brown. Add the zucchini and continue to cook for about 5 minutes, until softened.
4. In a large bowl, whisk the eggs until frothy. Season with salt and pepper.
5. Stir the ham and zucchini into the eggs. Add the chopped parsley and mix until well combined.
6. Pour the mixture into the prepared baking dish. Sprinkle the Asiago cheese evenly over the top and bake for 20—25 minutes, until the eggs are set.
7. Allow to rest for about 5 minutes before serving.

- - - - - - - - - - - - -
Zucchini is an excellent source of dietary fiber and contains high amounts of potassium, an important electrolyte that can help to reduce blood pressure.

NUTRITION FACTS (PER SERVING)

Total Carbohydrates: 3g	Dietary Fiber: 1g	Net Carbs: 2g
Protein: 15g	Total Fat: 12g	Calories: 182

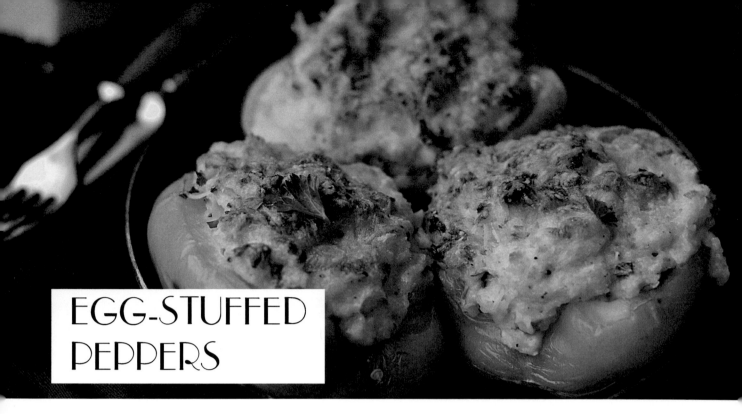

EGG-STUFFED PEPPERS

 5 minutes   **45 minutes**   **4**

INGREDIENTS

- » 4 yellow bell peppers, halved lengthwise and seeded
- » 5 large eggs
- » 1 cup shredded cheddar cheese
- » 4 slices bacon, cooked and crumbled
- » ¼ cup heavy cream
- » ¼ cup chopped frozen spinach, thawed
- » 3 green onions, chopped
- » Sea salt and pepper to taste

DIRECTIONS

1. Preheat oven to 350°F.
2. In a medium bowl, whisk the eggs and heavy cream together until frothy. Add the sliced green onions, spinach, half of the shredded cheese and bacon. Mix until well combined and season with salt and pepper.
3. Place the bell pepper halves in a lightly greased baking dish and divide the egg mixture between the peppers. Sprinkle with the remaining cheese.
4. Cover with foil and bake for 45 minutes, until the eggs are set.
5. Serve immediately.

- - - - - - - -

Bell peppers contain almost twice the daily recommended intake of vitamin C as well as hearty dose of antioxidants which benefit your immune system and help to keep your cells healthy.

NUTRITION FACTS (PER SERVING)

Total Carbohydrates: 10g	Dietary Fiber: 3g	Net Carbs: 7g
Protein: 23g	Total Fat: 19g	Calories: 273

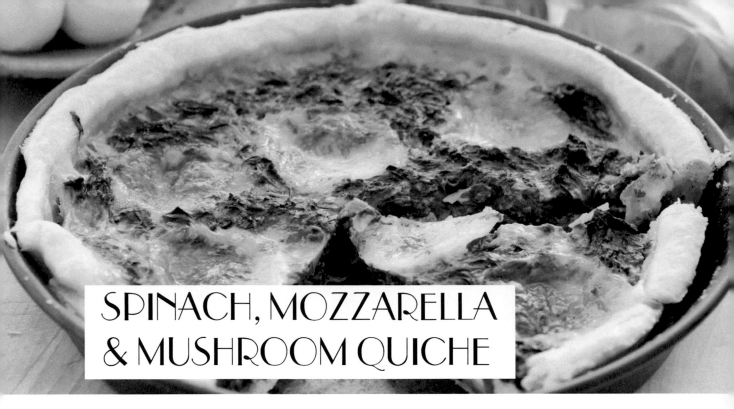

SPINACH, MOZZARELLA & MUSHROOM QUICHE

 5 minutes   **50 minutes** 👤 **6**

INGREDIENTS

» 1 (10 ounce) box frozen spinach, thawed and drained
» 2 (4 ounce) cans sliced mushrooms, drained
» 1 cup shredded mozzarella cheese
» ⅓ cup grated Parmesan cheese
» 6 large eggs
» ½ cup heavy cream
» ½ cup water
» ½ teaspoon garlic powder
» Sea salt and pepper to taste

DIRECTIONS

1. Preheat the oven to 350°F. Grease a 9-inch pie pan.
2. Evenly spread the thawed and drained spinach into the bottom of the pie pan. Top with the mushroom slices.
3. Whisk the eggs together with the heavy cream and water. Mix in the parmesan cheese, garlic powder, salt, and pepper.
4. Pour the egg mixture into the pan.
5. Sprinkle with mozzarella cheese and bake for 40—50 minutes, until the center is set and the edges are golden brown.
6. Remove from oven and allow to cool for 5—10 minutes. Slice and serve!

I ditched the carb-laden crust in this quiche recipe making the cooking process easier and the result just as delicious. This versatile recipe is a great way to use up whatever vegetables and cheeses you have on hand.

NUTRITION FACTS (PER SERVING)

Total Carbohydrates: 5g	Dietary Fiber: 1g	Net Carbs: 4g
Protein: 12g	Total Fat: 15g	Calories: 199

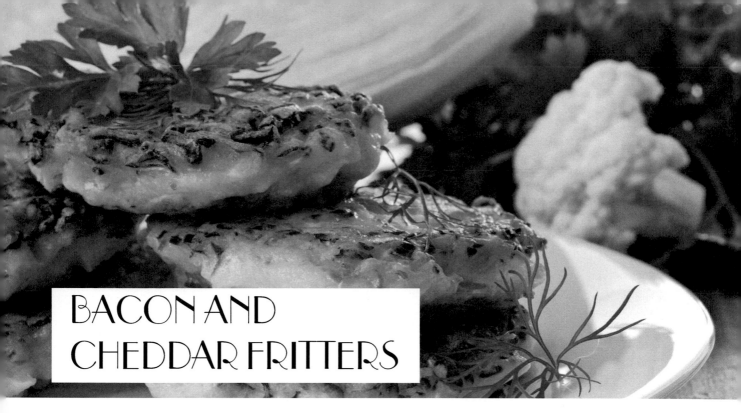

BACON AND CHEDDAR FRITTERS

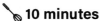 10 minutes 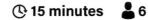 15 minutes   6

INGREDIENTS

» ⅔ cup cooked and crumbled bacon
» 1 ½ cups grated cheddar cheese
» 1 medium head cauliflower
» 3 large eggs
» 3 tablespoons coconut flour
» 2 cloves garlic, minced
» Sea salt and pepper to taste
» Coconut oil for the pan

DIRECTIONS

1. Chop the cauliflower into ½-inch pieces and steam for about 10—15 minutes, until soft. Drain well and mash with a fork or potato masher, pressing to release as much liquid as possible.
2. Transfer the cauliflower to a large bowl. Add the eggs, cheese, bacon, garlic, and coconut flour. Season with salt and pepper and mix well.
3. Heat a large skillet over medium heat and add about a tablespoon of coconut oil.
4. Form the cauliflower mixture into flat patties, using about 2—3 tablespoons per patty.
5. Once the pan is hot, add a few of the patties and cook for 3—5 minutes, until browned on the bottom. Flip carefully and cook another 3—5 minutes.
6. Remove to a paper towel-lined plate and repeat with the remaining patties.
7. Serve hot.

One serving of cauliflower contains 77% of your daily recommended amount of vitamin C. It's also a good source of fiber, potassium, and protein, believe it or not!

NUTRITION FACTS (PER SERVING)

Total Carbohydrates: 5g	Dietary Fiber: 2g	Net Carbs: 3g
Protein: 13g	Total Fat: 16g	Calories: 223

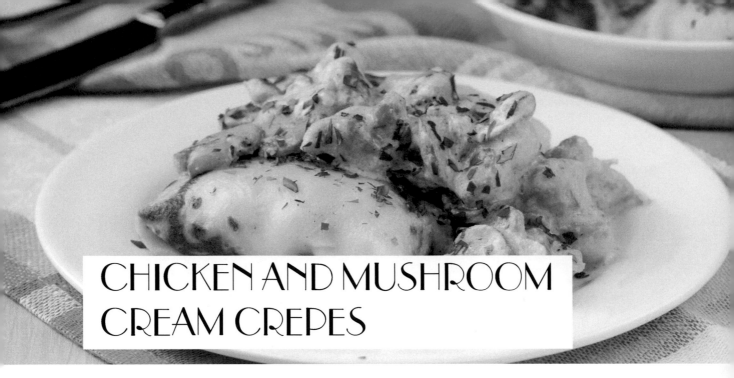

CHICKEN AND MUSHROOM CREAM CREPES

 10 minutes   **25 minutes**   👤 **4**

INGREDIENTS

» 1 boneless, skinless chicken breast, cut into ½-inch pieces
» 1 cup sliced mushrooms
» 2 cups heavy cream
» 4 large eggs
» 1 yellow onion, thinly sliced
» 4 slices bacon, cooked and chopped
» Sea salt and pepper to taste
» Olive oil for the pan
» Optional garnish: chopped parsley and/or chives

DIRECTIONS

1. Whisk the eggs together with about a tablespoon of heavy cream and season with salt and pepper.
2. Heat a small pan over medium heat and add a bit of olive oil to it.
3. Pour approximately ½ cup of the egg mixture to the pan and swirl to evenly coat the pan.
4. Once the eggs have set, flip and cook for about 1 minute. Transfer to a paper towel and repeat 3 times with the remaining egg mixture.
5. In a large pan, sautè the chicken, onions, and mushrooms together until the chicken is cooked through. Season with salt and pepper.
6. Stir in the bacon and the heavy cream. Cook about 3—4 minutes, until slightly thickened.
7. Divide most the chicken mixture between the 4 egg crepes, fold, and top with the remaining cream.
8. Serve and enjoy!

- - - - - - - - - - - - - -

For thousands of years, mushrooms have been celebrated as a powerful source for nutrients. They are a good source of B vitamins, which play an important role in the nervous system. They also contain high amounts of selenium, a mineral that is important to the immune system.

NUTRITION FACTS (PER SERVING)

Total Carbohydrates: 5g	Dietary Fiber: 1g	Net Carbs: 4g
Protein: 29g	Total Fat: 43g	Calories: 518

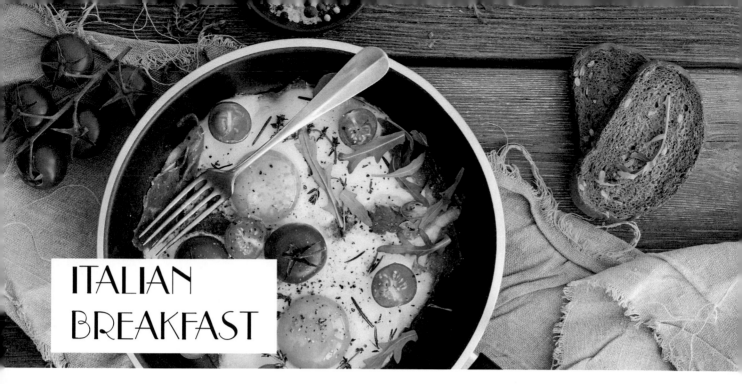

ITALIAN BREAKFAST

 5 minutes   🕐 **12 minutes**   👤 **4**

INGREDIENTS

- » 4 large eggs
- » 4 slices prosciutto ham
- » 12 cherry tomatoes, halved
- » 2 cloves garlic, minced
- » 1 cup rocket lettuce
- » 4 tablespoons of butter
- » Sea salt and black pepper to taste

DIRECTIONS

1. Heat 2 tablespoons of butter in a large skillet on a medium-high heat.
2. Crack and fry the eggs, preferably sunny side up, until the edges are golden (usually around 3—4 minutes). Remove from the pan and set aside for the moment.
3. Add the remaining butter, then add the garlic to the skillet and sautè until it begins to turn golden brown.
4. Add the cherry tomatoes and sautè for 3—4 minutes.
5. Layer the prosciutto and rocket lettuce on top of the tomatoes. Top with the precooked eggs.
6. Cover and allow everything to warm through for 2—3 minutes.
7. Season with additional salt and pepper, if desired, and serve immediately.

NUTRITION FACTS (PER SERVING)

| Total Carbohydrates: 5g | Dietary Fiber: 3g | Net Carbs: 2g |
| Protein: 11g | Total Fat: 19g | Calories: 228 |

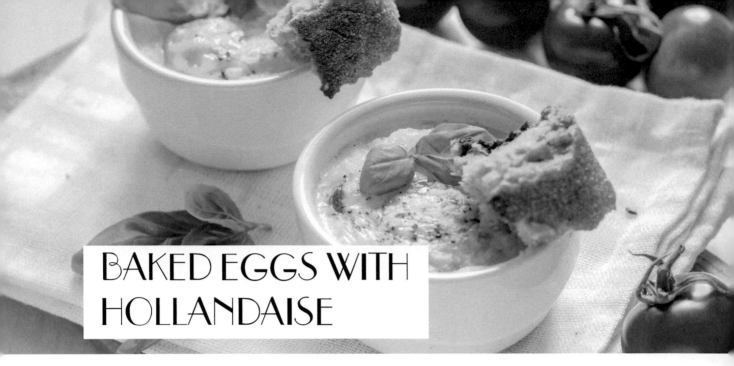

BAKED EGGS WITH HOLLANDAISE

 10 minutes   20 minutes   👤 4

INGREDIENTS

» 4 strips of bacon, chopped
» 2 cups baby spinach or kale
» 8 large eggs
» Optional garnish: fresh basil

Hollandaise Sauce

» 2 egg yolks
» ¼ cup butter, melted
» 1 tablespoon lemon juice
» ¼ teaspoon salt

DIRECTIONS

1. To prepare the hollandaise sauce: In a high speed blender, blend the egg yolks with the lemon juice and salt.
2. Slowly pour the melted butter into the blender while it's running. Blend for about 30 seconds, until thickened. Pour into a small bowl set over a sauce pan of simmering water to keep warm until ready to use.
3. For the baked eggs: Preheat oven to 400°F. Position the rack in the top third of the oven.
4. Heat a large skillet over medium heat. Cook the bacon until crisp.
5. Add the greens and sautè until wilted. Divide the mixture evenly between 4 large ramekins or gratin dishes.
6. Gently crack 2 eggs onto the filling of each ramekin. Place on a baking sheet and into the oven for 10—12 minutes, until the white is set, but the yolk is still runny.
7. Drizzle with hollandaise sauce, garnish with fresh basil, if desired, and serve immediately.
8. I cannot help but to serve this dish with a couple of 'soldiers'. The yolks are great for dipping a couple of sticks of low-carb bread into.

Hollandaise sauce is a simple emulsion of egg yolk and butter that is widely used in French cooking. It adds a creamy richness to the eggs in this recipe. If you'd like to spice it up a bit, try adding a pinch of cayenne pepper to it before blending.

NUTRITION FACTS (PER SERVING)

Total Carbohydrates: 2g	Dietary Fiber: 1g	Net Carbs: 1g
Protein: 24g	Total Fat: 34g	Calories: 411

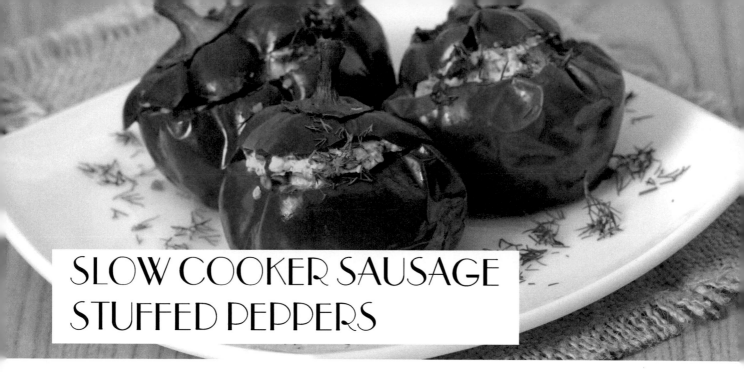

SLOW COOKER SAUSAGE STUFFED PEPPERS

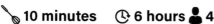 **10 minutes**   🕐 **6 hours** 👤 **4**

INGREDIENTS

- » 1 pound Italian sausage
- » 4 bell peppers
- » ½ head of cauliflower
- » 1 (8 ounce) can tomato paste
- » 1 small yellow onion, diced
- » 3 garlic cloves, minced
- » 2 teaspoons oregano
- » Sea salt and pepper to taste

DIRECTIONS

1. Cut the tops off of the bell peppers and discard the seeds. Save the tops.
2. Grate the cauliflower into "œrice" with a cheese grater or food processor and transfer to a large mixing bowl.
3. Add the minced garlic, oregano, and onion. Mix well to combine.
4. Add the sausage and tomato paste to the cauliflower mixture and mix well with your hands. Season with salt and pepper.
5. Evenly divide the sausage mixture between the peppers. Cover each pepper with their tops and gently place into your slow cooker.
6. Cook on low for 6 hours.
7. Serve and enjoy!

Bell peppers have quite a bit going for them. They're low in calories, high in fiber, and an excellent source of vitamins A and C.

NUTRITION FACTS (PER SERVING)

Total Carbohydrates: 18g	Dietary Fiber: 6g	Net Carbs: 12g
Protein: 27g	Total Fat: 33g	Calories: 485

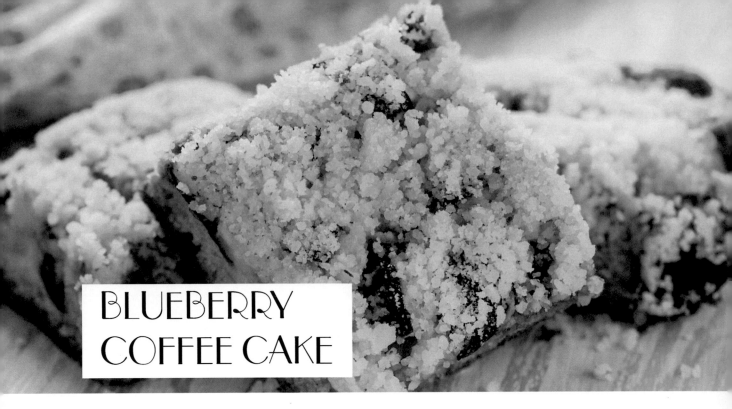

BLUEBERRY COFFEE CAKE

 15 minutes   🕐 **30 minutes**   👤 **6**

INGREDIENTS

» 1 cup fresh or frozen blueberries (or other berry of choice)
» 4 large eggs, separated
» ½ cup coconut flour
» ¼ cup coconut oil
» ¼ cup sugar substitute
» 2 teaspoons vanilla extract
» ¼ teaspoon baking soda
» 1 teaspoon cream of tartar

Topping
» ¼ cup coconut sugar
» ¼ cup coconut oil
» 2 tablespoons coconut flour
» ½ teaspoon cinnamon

DIRECTIONS

1. Preheat oven to 350°F. Prepare an 8x8 baking pan with non-stick spray.
2. In a large bowl, combine the egg whites and cream of tartar. Whisk until stiff peaks form.
3. In another bowl, cream together the sugar substitute and coconut oil. Mix in the egg yolks.
4. Slowly stir in the coconut flour, vanilla, and baking soda. Mix until just combined.
5. Gently fold the egg whites into the batter. Pour into the prepared pan. Evenly scatter the blueberries on top.
6. In a small bowl, mix the ingredients for the topping.
7. Spread the mixture over the batter.
8. Bake for 30 minutes, or until a toothpick inserted comes out clean.
9. Allow to cool to room temperature before cutting into squares.

Coconut flour is a versatile kitchen staple that's popular in the keto community. It's high in fiber and a great source of heart-healthy fats.

NUTRITION FACTS (PER SERVING)

Total Carbohydrates: 6g	Dietary Fiber: 2g	Net Carbs: 4g
Protein: 6g	Total Fat: 26g	Calories: 270

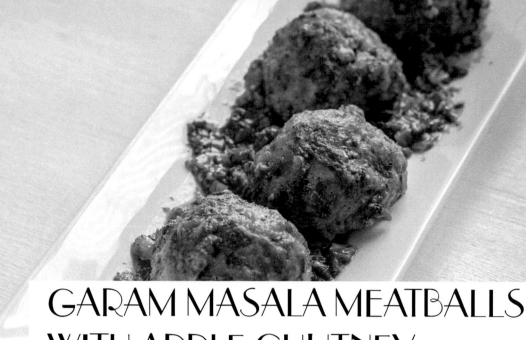

GARAM MASALA MEATBALLS WITH APPLE CHUTNEY

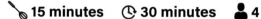 15 minutes   30 minutes   4

INGREDIENTS

For the Meatballs

» ½ pound lean ground pork
» 1 teaspoon onion powder
» 1 teaspoon salt
» 1 teaspoon garam masala

For the Apple Chutney

» 2 medium tart apples (such as Granny Smith)
» ¼ cup raisins
» 2 tablespoons butter
» ½ teaspoon garam masala
» 1 tablespoon maple syrup
» 2 tablespoons water
» 1 tablespoon apple cider vinegar

DIRECTIONS

1. Preheat oven to 400°F. Line a baking sheet with parchment paper.
2. In a large bowl, combine all of the meatball ingredients. Mix well with hands.
3. Portion into small balls and bake for about 15—20 minutes, until cooked through.
4. To prepare the chutney: Combine all of the ingredients into a medium saucepan over medium heat.
5. Bring to a simmer, cover, and allow to cook for 6—8 minutes, stirring occasionally.
6. Mash the chutney with a potato masher or fork until few chunks remain.
7. Top the meatballs with the chutney and enjoy.

Garam masala is an aromatic blend of ground spices common in Indian cuisine. It can be found in the international aisle of most grocery stores.

NUTRITION FACTS (PER SERVING)

Total Carbohydrates: 18g	Dietary Fiber: 3g	Net Carbs: 15g
Protein: 16g	Total Fat: 12g	Calories: 249

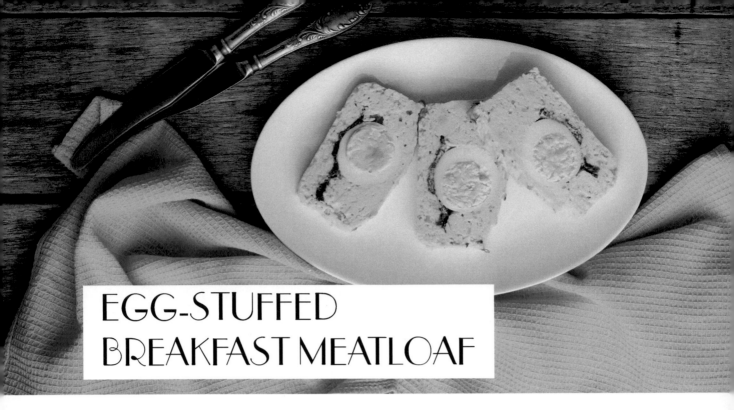

EGG-STUFFED BREAKFAST MEATLOAF

🥄 15 minutes   🕐 35 minutes   👤 6

INGREDIENTS

- » 4 hardboiled eggs, peeled
- » 1 cup baby spinach or kale
- » 1 ½ pounds ground pork
- » 1 teaspoon smoked paprika
- » 1 teaspoon fennel seeds
- » ½ teaspoon salt
- » ½ teaspoon pepper
- » ½ teaspoon sage
- » ¼ teaspoon cayenne pepper

DIRECTIONS

1. Preheat oven to 400°F. Prepare a 9x5 inch loaf pan with non-stick spray.
2. In a large mixing bowl, combine the ground pork with the spices and mix well with hands.
3. Place a thin layer of pork in the bottom of the prepared pan.
4. Line the baby spinach down the center of the pan and top with the hard boiled eggs.
5. Place the remaining pork on top and press gently.
6. Bake for 35 minutes, or until golden brown.
7. Allow to cool for 5—10 minutes. Slice and serve.

Meatloaf doesn't have to be just for dinner. This savory breakfast meatloaf is a unique spin on eggs and sausage. Individual slices can be wrapped tightly in plastic wrap and stored in the freezer for several weeks.

NUTRITION FACTS (PER SERVING)

Total Carbohydrates: 0g	Dietary Fiber: 2g	Net Carbs: 0g
Protein: 33g	Total Fat: 7g	Calories: 204g

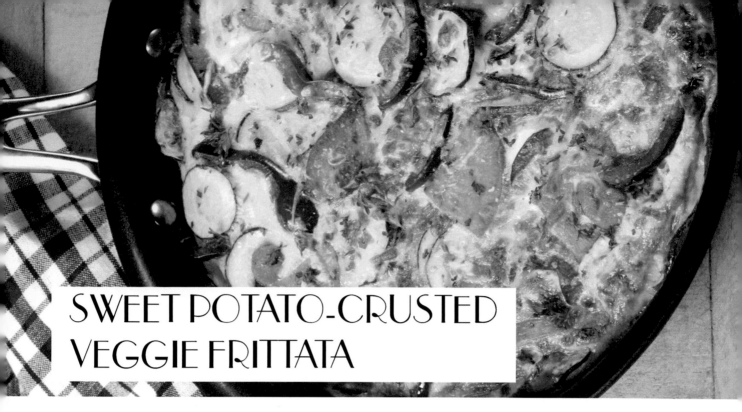

SWEET POTATO-CRUSTED VEGGIE FRITTATA

🥄 **15 minutes**   🕐 **60 minutes**   👤 **6**

INGREDIENTS

» 2 sweet potatoes, peeled and very thinly sliced
» 1 medium zucchini, sliced
» 1 bell pepper, sliced
» 2 cups baby spinach
» 3 bacon slices, cooked and crumbled (reserve about 1 tablespoon of the fat)
» 1 small onion, sliced
» 5 eggs, beaten
» 2 tablespoons olive oil
» 2 cloves garlic, minced
» Sea salt and pepper to taste

DIRECTIONS

1. Preheat oven to 400°F.
2. Toss the sweet potato slices with olive oil and season with salt and pepper.
3. Arrange the slices in a 9" pie dish to form a crust for the quiche. Bake for 15—20 minutes.
4. While the crust bakes, add the reserved bacon fat to a large skillet over medium heat.
5. Sautè the garlic, zucchini, bell pepper and onion until translucent. Add the spinach and cook until wilted. Remove from heat.
6. Once the sweet potatoes are done, lower the heat to 375°F.
7. Layer the spinach mixture into the crust, top with the beaten eggs and crumbled bacon. Season with salt and pepper and bake for 30—35 minutes, until the eggs are set.
8. Serve warm.

Eating deep orange-colored fruits and vegetables, such as sweet potatoes, is associated with lower risk of coronary heart disease. A good reason to include them in your regular diet!

NUTRITION FACTS (PER SERVING)

Total Carbohydrates: 14g	Dietary Fiber: 3g	Net Carbs: 11g
Protein: 9g	Total Fat: 12g	Calories: 212

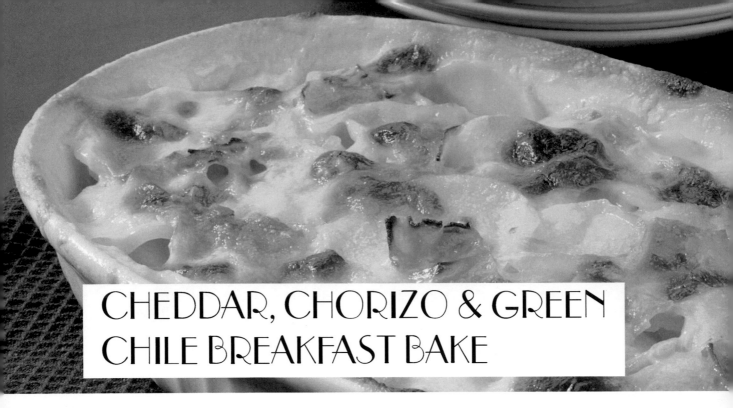

CHEDDAR, CHORIZO & GREEN CHILE BREAKFAST BAKE

🥄 **15 minutes**   🕐 **45 minutes**   👤 **6**

INGREDIENTS

» 1 pound chorizo sausage
» 1 (8 ounce) can green chilies
» 1 cup shredded cheddar cheese
» 1 yellow onion, diced
» ½ head cauliflower
» 4 eggs, beaten
» ½ teaspoon garlic powder
» Sea salt and pepper to taste
» Optional garnish: sliced green onions

DIRECTIONS

1. Preheat oven to 375°F. Grease a 9x13 glass baking dish with olive oil.
2. In a skillet over medium heat, cook the chorizo and onion until golden brown.
3. Add the chilies to the pan and mix well. Transfer to a large mixing bowl and allow to cool slightly.
4. Shred the cauliflower into "rice" using a food processor or cheese grater. Add to the bowl.
5. Stir in the beaten eggs and half of the cheese. Season with salt, pepper, and garlic salt. Pour into the prepared dish. Top with the remaining cheese.
6. Bake for 45 minutes, until the eggs are set and cheese is golden brown.
7. Let rest for 5 minutes. Top with green onions, if desired. Serve!

Chorizo is a pork sausage that is heavily seasoned with paprika and other spices. It can be found in most grocery stores, but regular breakfast sausage can be substituted, if it's not available in your area.

NUTRITION FACTS (PER SERVING)

Total Carbohydrates: 22g	Dietary Fiber: 12g	Net Carbs: 10g
Protein: 23g	Total Fat: 27g	Calories: 430

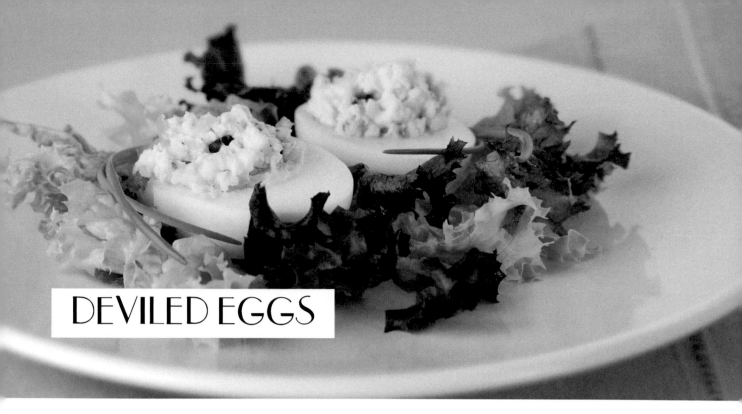

DEVILED EGGS

 15 minutes   10 minutes   🧑 4

INGREDIENTS

- » 8 hardboiled eggs, peeled and sliced in half
- » 1 tablespoon mayonnaise
- » 1 teaspoon Dijon mustard
- » 1 tablespoon heavy cream
- » 1 tablespoon olive oil
- » 1 clove garlic, minced
- » 1 tablespoon green onion, minced
- » 1 teaspoon lemon juice
- » 2 tablespoons parsley, roughly chopped

DIRECTIONS

1. Gently remove the yolks from the hard boiled eggs and place in a medium bowl. Place the whites on a serving tray.
2. Add the mayonnaise, mustard, heavy cream, olive oil, garlic, green onion, lemon juice, and parsley.
3. Mash everything together until a thick paste forms. Spoon the mixture back into the egg whites.
4. Serve over a bed of salad greens.

The concept of deviled eggs began in Ancient Rome although the name is an 18th century invention. The word "deviled" was used to describe highly seasoned fried or boiled dishes.

NUTRITION FACTS (PER SERVING)

Total Carbohydrates: 2g	Dietary Fiber: 0g	Net Carbs: 2g
Protein: 11g	Total Fat: 19g	Calories: 217

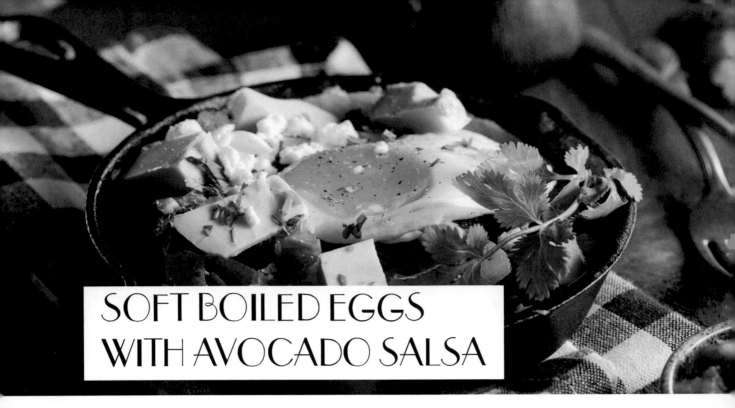

SOFT BOILED EGGS WITH AVOCADO SALSA

 15 minutes   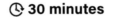 **30 minutes**   **4**

INGREDIENTS

- » 8 large eggs
- » 1 avocado, diced
- » 1 cup cherry tomatoes, quartered
- » ¼ cup red onion, diced
- » ½ cup cilantro, roughly chopped
- » ½ a jalapeño, minced
- » ¼ cup feta cheese
- » ½ teaspoon sea salt
- » Juice of 1 lime

DIRECTIONS

1. To prepare the avocado salsa: Combine everything but the eggs in a medium bowl and mix well. Cover and refrigerate until ready to serve.
2. To soft boil the eggs: Fill a medium saucepan with water and bring to a boil. Reduce heat to a simmer and add the eggs to the pot.
3. Cook 5 minutes for a runny yolk, or 7 minutes for a soft-set yolk.
4. Remove from heat and run the eggs under cold water for about 1 minute, or until cool enough to peel.
5. Gently peel the eggs and plate with a big scoop of the avocado salsa. Enjoy!

Soft boiled egg tip: Work in batches of 4 eggs at a time to avoid overcrowding the saucepan. Be sure to set a timer, they can go from soft boiled to hard boiled very quickly, if you're not paying attention.

NUTRITION FACTS (PER SERVING)

Total Carbohydrates: 8g	Dietary Fiber: 4g	Net Carbs: 4g
Protein: 13g	Total Fat: 19g	Calories: 240

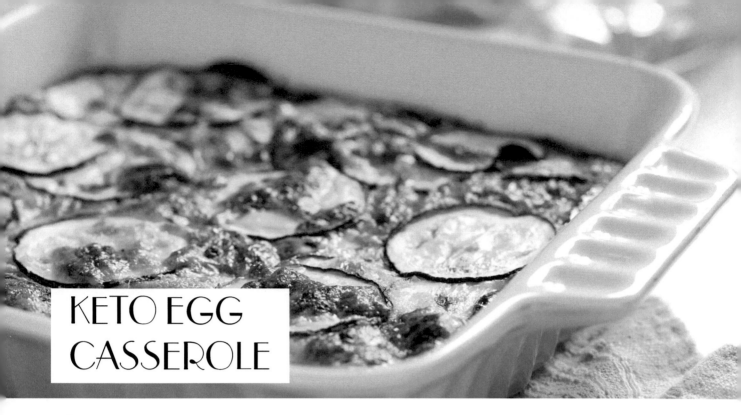

KETO EGG CASSEROLE

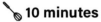 **10 minutes**   **30 minutes** 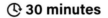 **6**

INGREDIENTS

- » 12 large eggs
- » 1 pound breakfast sausage
- » 1 zucchini, thinly sliced
- » ½ red onion, diced
- » ½ green pepper, diced
- » 1 cup half & half
- » ½ cup shredded cheddar cheese
- » ¼ teaspoon thyme
- » Sea salt and pepper to taste
- » Optional garnish: chopped fresh basil leaves

DIRECTIONS

1. Preheat oven to 350°F. Prepare an 8x8 baking dish with non-stick spray.
2. In a large skillet over medium heat, brown the sausage.
3. Once the sausage is cooked through, add the onions, peppers, and zucchini. Cook until tender. Remove from heat.
4. In a large bowl, whisk the eggs until frothy. Season with salt, pepper, and thyme.
5. Add the vegetables to the eggs and pour into the prepared baking dish. Sprinkle evenly with the shredded cheese.
6. Bake for 30 minutes, until the eggs are set.
7. Garnish with chopped basil, if desired and serve.

This simple recipe can be adapted any way you like. Get creative and throw in whatever add-ins you'd like! Cheese, hot peppers, and black olives are all great choices. Add a fried egg on top for decoration when having friends over.

NUTRITION FACTS (PER SERVING)

Total Carbohydrates: 4g	Dietary Fiber: 1g	Net Carbs: 3g
Protein: 30g	Total Fat: 38g	Calories: 478

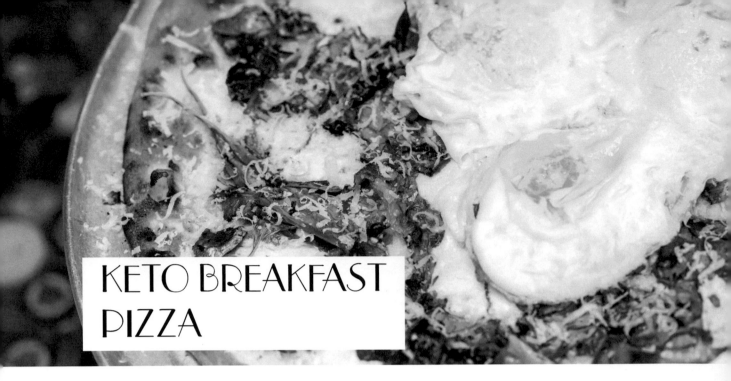

KETO BREAKFAST PIZZA

 10 minutes   30 minutes   👤 6

INGREDIENTS

Pizza Dough

» ½ cup coconut flour
» 3 eggs
» 1 cup canned coconut milk
» 1 teaspoon onion powder
» 1 teaspoon garlic powder
» ½ teaspoon baking powder
» ½ teaspoon baking soda
» ¼ teaspoon dried basil
» ¼ teaspoon dried oregano

Pizza Toppings

» 9 eggs, beaten
» ½ pound breakfast sausage
» 1 red onion, thinly sliced
» 6 garlic cloves, minced
» 8 sun-dried tomatoes
» 2 tablespoons olive oil
» 1 cup baby spinach, roughly chopped

DIRECTIONS

1. Preheat oven to 425°F.
2. In a large bowl, combine the coconut flour with the baking powder, baking soda, and spices.
3. Add the coconut milk and eggs and mix well. Set aside to rest for 5 minutes. Dough will be very soft — more like batter.
4. Line a baking sheet with parchment paper and spread the pizza dough over it evenly. Bake for 25 minutes, or until golden brown.
5. In a large skillet over medium heat, brown the breakfast sausage until golden brown. Transfer to a plate.
6. Add the olive oil to the pan and cook the onion, garlic, and sun-dried tomatoes until softened.
7. For the eggs, you can either add them to the pan and scramble together with the other ingredients, or fry them and put them on top after (for presentation purposes, I prefer to fry them).
8. Top the pizza crust evenly with the eggs and sausage.
9. Place back in the oven and bake for 5—7 minutes. Remove from oven, slice, and serve.

- - - - - - - - -

Following a keto diet doesn't mean giving up the foods that you love, especially pizza! This recipe is sure to please kids and adults alike.

NUTRITION FACTS (PER SERVING)

Total Carbohydrates: 11g	Dietary Fiber: 5g	Net Carbs: 6g
Protein: 22g	Total Fat: 35g	Calories: 444

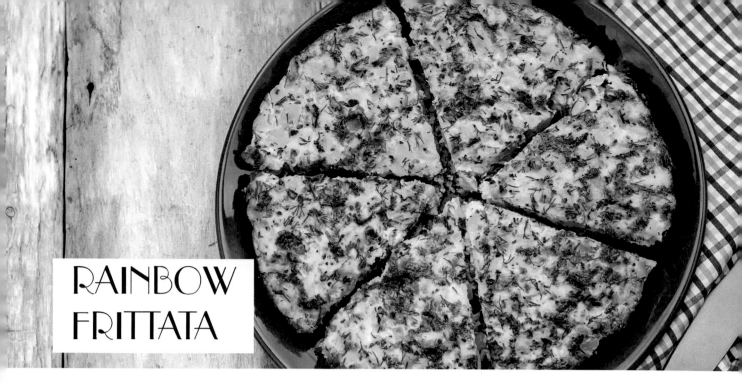

RAINBOW FRITTATA

 10 minutes   **20 minutes**   🧍 **6**

INGREDIENTS

- » 8 eggs
- » 1 small red onion, thinly sliced
- » 1 small head of broccoli, cut into small florets
- » 2 cups baby spinach or kale
- » 2 tomatoes, thinly sliced
- » 1 large carrot, grated
- » 3 cloves garlic, minced
- » ¼ cup feta cheese
- » Sea salt and pepper to taste
- » 2 tablespoons olive oil

DIRECTIONS

1. Preheat oven to 350°F. Prepare a 9-inch pie plate with non-stick spray.
2. Heat the olive oil in a large skillet over medium-high heat.
3. Sautè the onions and garlic until translucent. Add the broccoli florets and reduce heat to medium-low. Cover and cook for 5 minutes, until the broccoli is tender.
4. Add the spinach and cook until slightly wilted.
5. Remove from heat and transfer to your prepared pie plate.
6. In a large bowl, whisk the eggs with the carrot and feta cheese. Season with salt and pepper and carefully pour over the vegetable mixture.
7. Top with the sliced tomatoes and bake for 20 minutes, or until the eggs are set.
8. Allow to rest for 10 minutes before slicing and serving.

This super easy veggie frittata makes a great breakfast, but is also delicious served over salad greens for a quick and healthy lunch.

NUTRITION FACTS (PER SERVING)

Total Carbohydrates: 8g	Dietary Fiber: 2g	Net Carbs: 6g
Protein: 10g	Total Fat: 12g	Calories: 175

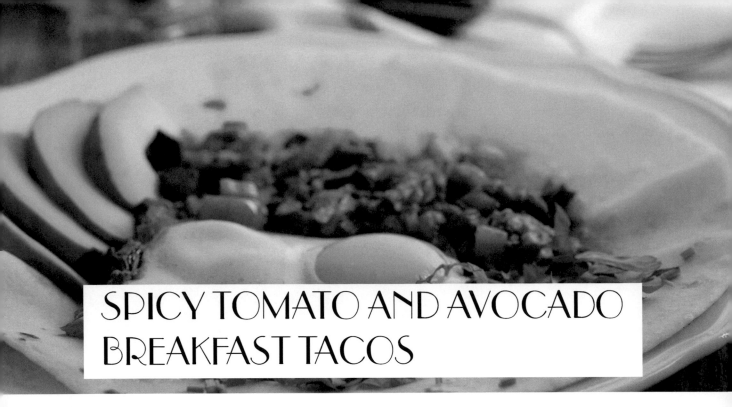

SPICY TOMATO AND AVOCADO BREAKFAST TACOS

 5 minutes   ⏱ 15 minutes   👤 4

INGREDIENTS

» 4 eggs
» 1 (10 ounce) can Ro-Tel tomatoes
» 1 ripe avocado, thinly sliced
» Sea salt and pepper
» ½ cup fresh cilantro, chopped
» 4 low-carb tortillas

DIRECTIONS

1. Preheat oven to 400°F. Spray a medium sized, ovenproof skillet with non-stick spray. (Cast iron works great.)
2. Pour the tomatoes into the skillet and place over medium heat.
3. Once almost all of the liquid has evaporated from the tomatoes, crack the eggs on top and season with salt and pepper.
4. Transfer the skillet to the oven and bake for 10—12 minutes, until the egg whites are set.
5. Serve each egg alongside sliced avocado and fresh cilantro, with a low-carb tortilla.

The high lycopene content of tomatoes protects the body from UV rays thus offering defense against skin cancer.

NUTRITION FACTS (PER SERVING)

Total Carbohydrates: 19g	Dietary Fiber: 11g	Net Carbs: 8g
Protein: 10g	Total Fat: 16g	Calories: 258

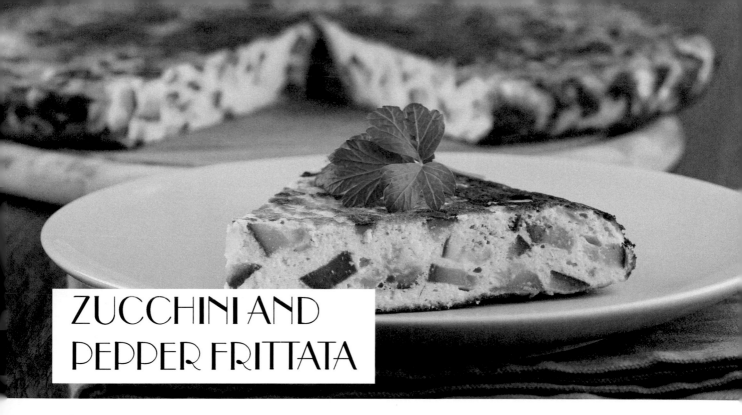

ZUCCHINI AND PEPPER FRITTATA

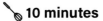 10 minutes 　　 🕐 25 minutes 　　 👤 6

INGREDIENTS

» 8 large eggs
» 2 medium zucchinis, thinly sliced
» 1 red onion, thinly sliced
» 2 green peppers, thinly sliced
» 2 cloves garlic, minced
» 2 tablespoons olive oil
» Sea salt and pepper to taste
» Optional topping: Pico de Gallo or salsa

DIRECTIONS

1. Preheat oven to 400°F.
2. Heat 1 tablespoon of olive oil in a 9-inch ovenproof pan. Add the onion, zucchini slices, bell pepper and garlic. Cook for about 5 minutes, until softened.
3. While the veggies cook, whisk the eggs with the salt and pepper in a large bowl.
4. Add the zucchini mixture to the eggs and mix well.
5. Heat the remaining tablespoon of olive oil in the pan and add the egg mixture. Cook over medium heat for 5 minutes.
6. Transfer pan to the oven and bake for 20 minutes, until the eggs are set.
7. Remove from oven; allow to cool for 10 minutes. Carefully flip onto a serving platter and slice into wedges.
8. Top with Pico de Gallo or salsa, if desired, and serve!

Zucchini has such a mild flavor that it can be adapted into just about any dish. They're low calorie, low carb, and add a healthy dose of fiber to this dish.

NUTRITION FACTS (PER SERVING)

Total Carbohydrates: 5g	Dietary Fiber: 1g	Net Carbs: 4g
Protein: 8g	Total Fat: 11g	Calories: 142

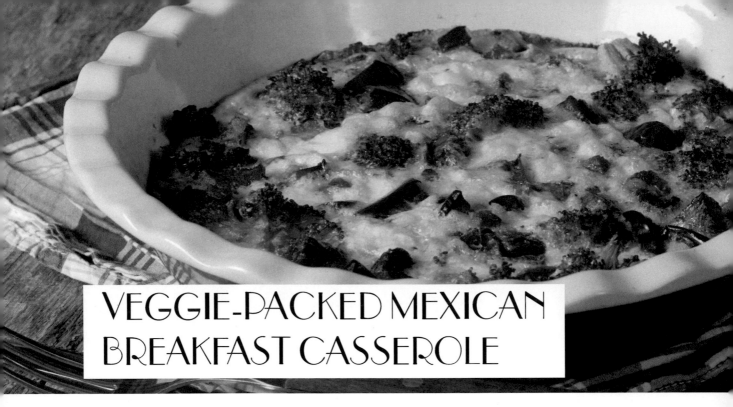

VEGGIE-PACKED MEXICAN BREAKFAST CASSEROLE

 10 minutes   25 minutes   👤 6

INGREDIENTS

» 8 eggs, beaten
» ½ cup broccoli florets
» ½ pound bacon
» 1 yellow onion, diced
» 1 red bell pepper, diced
» 8 ounces mushrooms, sliced
» 1 sweet potato, peeled and diced
» 2 tablespoons taco seasoning
» Garnish: guacamole, salsa, and fresh cilantro

DIRECTIONS

1. Cook the bacon in a skillet until crispy. Set aside. Crumble once cooled.
2. In the same skillet, cook the onions until translucent.
3. Transfer the crumbled bacon, onions, sweet potato, bell pepper, mushrooms, broccoli florets and eggs to a slow cooker. Stir to combine.
4. Sprinkle with taco seasoning and mix well.
5. Cook on low for 6 hours.
6. Scoop into serving bowls, top with guacamole, salsa, and/or fresh cilantro.

You can use packaged taco seasoning for this recipe or make your own by combing the following spices: 2 tablespoons chili powder, ½ teaspoon garlic powder, ½ teaspoon onion powder, ½ teaspoon red pepper flakes, ½ teaspoon oregano, 1 teaspoon paprika, 1 tablespoon cumin, 2 teaspoons salt, 2 teaspoons pepper.

NUTRITION FACTS (PER SERVING)

Total Carbohydrates: 12g	Dietary Fiber: 3g	Net Carbs: 9g
Protein: 24g	Total Fat: 25g	Calories: 360

BONUS KETO SWEET EATS SERIES

I am delighted you have chosen my book to help you start or continue on your keto journey. Temptation by sweet treats can knock you off course so, to help you stay on the keto track, I am pleased to offer you three mini ebooks from my 'Keto Sweet Eats Series', completely free of charge! These three mini ebooks cover how to make everything from keto chocolate cake to keto ice cream to keto fat bombs so you don't have to feel like you are missing out, whatever the occasion.

Simply visit the link below to get your free copy of all three mini ebooks...

http://geni.us/breakbonus

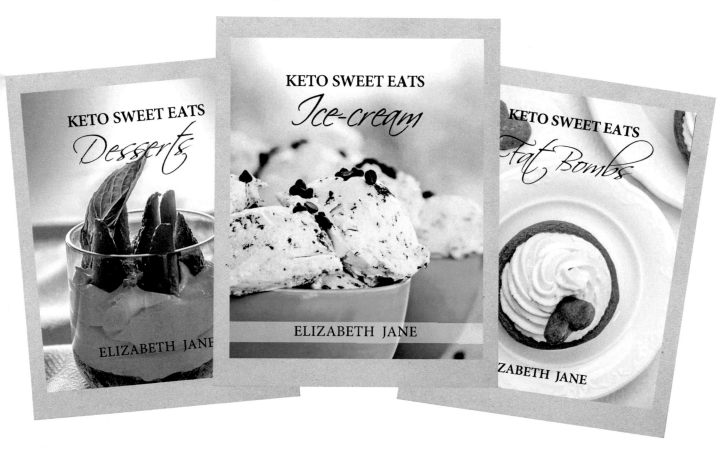

Made in the USA
Middletown, DE
06 March 2018